PRIMAL BODY—
PRIMAL MIND

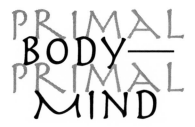

PRIMAL BODY—PRIMAL MIND

EMPOWER YOUR TOTAL HEALTH THE WAY EVOLUTION INTENDED (...AND DIDN'T)

NORA T. GEDGAUDAS, CNS, CNT

Primal Body—Primal Mind Publishing
Portland, Oregon

Primal Body—Primal Mind Publishing
(An assumed business name of Northwest Neurofeedback, Inc., an Oregon corporation)
P.O. Box 10766
Portland, OR 97296-0766
www.PrimalBody-PrimalMind.com

ISBN: 978-0-9821841-0-3
Library of Congress Control Number: 2008939931

Front cover: Paleolithic cave painting from Lascaux, France.
Photo by RALPH MORSE. Used by permission from Time-Life
    (Getty Images)
Author photo by ROSEMARY RAGUSA of Mon Amour Photography
    (www.monamourphotography.com)
Cover design by KIRK KRISTLIBAS of Avalonik Society Media
    (www.avaloniksocietymedia.org)
Interior design by JENNIFER OMNER of ALL Publications
    (www.ALLPublications.com)

Disclaimer:
The information in this book is not meant to diagnose, prescribe or treat any illness. Please discuss any changes you wish to make to your medical treatment with a qualified health provider.

For Lisa, without whose tireless dedication and support this book would not have been possible. Also, this book is for all those in my life who have relentlessly supported me, my heart and my work. You have my eternal love and gratitude.

And finally, for our ancestors—who hold an important key for all of us to the future of our survival.

The writer is fully aware that his message is not orthodox; but since our orthodox theories have not saved us we may have to readjust them to bring them into harmony with Nature's laws. Nature must be obeyed, not orthodoxy.

—WESTON A. PRICE
from *Nutrition and Physical Degeneration* (1939)

CONTENTS

PART 1: PRIMAL BODY

PART 2: PRIMAL MIND

PART 3: PARADISE LOST

ILLUSTRATIONS

FOREWORD

Every so often, you encounter a gem among the dross competing for your attention. Such is the case with *Primal Body—Primal Mind,* written by Nora Gedgaudas.

This book is a nutritional treasure map leading to optimal wellness the way nature intended. The author has outlined and detailed a thorough documentation of nutritional principles and has linked them directly to evolutionary history. More important, she has provided direct guidelines for shopping and eating in ways that eliminate a host of physiological and mental disorders and restore followers to the natural condition of health and wellness that results from eating as we were biologically designed.

Gedgaudas' book is loaded with facts, numbers and startling revelations, but it is also replete with understandable explanations and solutions tied to everyday actions and changes that anyone can make. Even if you read it without any intention of changing your diet, *Primal Body—Primal Mind* is a non-fictional excursion into the realm of biology, politics and self-care that you will never get from formal academic education. It is worth reading as a short, comprehensible course in the biochemistry of behavior and of consumerism. Her approach to the Paleolithic dietary habits that have sustained humans without pills or potions for millennia stands in stark and clean defiance against the nonsense peddled for our allegiance and dollars so relentlessly.

Gedgaudas teaches things that your mother should have, and she does so without nagging or sermonizing. Her writing is eloquent, factual and straightforward, and she provides many practical tips, including Web sites and other resources. Her arguments and data are scientifically documented, and the book is well organized and easily referenced.

Reading Gedgaudas' jewel might make you a bit sheepish about how you've been duped by so many commercial interests, including the diet and publishing industries. Quickly, however, you will be grateful for her leadership out of the wilderness of illness and digestive trickery that so easily nickel-and-dimes us away from truly feeling good, and maintaining our high quality of life.

In reading *Primal Body—Primal Mind,* it becomes obvious that Gedgaudas cares for herself and for others. I know this firsthand, since Nora is a colleague engaged in the clinical practice of EEG Neurotherapy. As a neuropsychologist with thirty years of experience and the author of a popular book on brain training and mental fitness, I endorse Nora's exemplary use of scientific techniques, and her reputation and expertise in the clinical care of people. She is among the elite professionals who can restore health and promote growth by harnessing nature's principles with effective care.

I have learned a lot from Nora and from *Primal Body—Primal Mind,* and I believe that this is "must" reading for anyone serious about healthcare and self-care.

MARK STEINBERG, PhD
Licensed Psychologist
Clinical Neuropsychologist
NBC Medical Consultant
Author of *ADD: The 20-Hour Solution*

PREFACE

As a clinical neurofeedback practitioner specializing in EEG bio-feedback (also known as neurotherapy, neuro-biofeedback, and brain training), I help individuals exercise or condition their brains in a way that allows for greater stability, enhanced cognitive functioning, and improved affect and ability to pay attention. It is a means of impacting both the regulation and functional dysregulation of a nervous system through a non-invasive and self-empowering process. Neurofeedback is best likened to highly-specialized "brain exercise." At its best, neurofeedback seems to restore a neurological flexibility, stress-coping capacity and a certain improved homeostasis that should be everyone's birthright. It can free one from self-imposed obstacles and allow the full flowering of human potential.

Using neurofeedback, I myself was freed from over thirty years of intractable depression that had not responded to *anything else.* The concomitant anxiety and panic attacks I experienced almost daily, too, became part of the past. It was a freedom and a liberation that has made me a devout practitioner of this miraculous form of brain training ever since. That was many years ago. The effect I have since witnessed in thousands of individuals has been so profound that, I am convinced, neurofeedback is the most powerful means available to facilitate permanent and positive changes in neurological functioning. It is the most rewarding work I can possibly imagine.

However, I have found individuals repeatedly plateauing in their process, simply hitting walls they couldn't seem to hurdle. Some experience inexplicable backslides or have difficulty getting their brains to move at all. What such experience has revealed to me, over and over, is that typically there seems to be an issue with diet, food sensitivity, endocrine dysfunction and/or severe nutritional deficiencies. Almost without exception, addressing these dietary issues allows the obstacles to be overcome, and healing improvements are then free to take place. Everything comes together far more efficiently. The brain and body simply have to have certain raw materials to work with in order to function properly. It is abundantly clear that all the brain-training in the world cannot create a nutrient where there is none or remove a problematic substance which does not belong.

My more than twenty-five years of background in the passionate, intricate study and application of nutritional science and, more recently, nutritional anthropology, served to beautifully cement and maintain my own neurotherapy results. Dietary intervention with clients has repeatedly provided a powerful solution to such dilemmas. Counseling my clients regarding diet, however, is something that proved to be time consuming and often overwhelming for all involved. As a believer in providing detailed education and not prescriptions, I found that there was simply too much information to convey and too little time to convey it. I was at a loss to recommend any single source of literature to provide answers to my clients, as no single source seemed adequate in its scope. I found myself spending untold time and money copying articles and pages from books and offering lengthy explanations. This arrangement was an enormous source of frustration for all involved.

As such, frustration became the mother of invention, and this book was born. In its infancy, this was little more than a five- or ten-page article, outlining basic principles and providing a few resources. With all the positive feedback, however, came more questions—lots of questions. I also realized that much of what I was providing as information was at times controversial and not voiced in the mainstream health-oriented mantras. I needed to provide more clear references and illustrate the solid foundations of the framework I was gradually building in writing. More and more information seemed important to add—either as clarification or as pertinent adjunct to these principles. The modest five or ten pages began to grow. Increasingly positive feedback and excellent clinical results ensued, and there were still more questions. Eventually the whole thing grew and evolved. This newly revised, substantially expanded and updated volume is the result.

Today I utilize this book, nutritional counseling and nutritional therapy with both my neurofeedback clients and with those solely interested in dietary help. The results have been overwhelmingly positive.

Many, many individuals have benefited profoundly from the information presented here. Tremendously positive and inspiring results have been reported. I have seen weight loss when it was needed; restored digestive health when nothing else worked; substantially improved blood chemistry reports; total liberation from food cravings and eating disorders—even addictions. I have also seen liberation from antidepressants, psychostimulants, and other types of medications; enhanced energy levels; improvements in mental clarity and affect; improved sustainability of attention; reduced anxieties and instabilities; and freedom from unnecessary dependence on gimmicks, gurus, and supplements. People are even reporting big savings on their grocery bills!

Most rewarding of all, I have come to see others become students of health themselves, no longer relying on controlling, confusing or contradictory advice from diet pundits and "dictocrats," to borrow a creative term coined by Sally Fallon. Utilizing sound, common-sense principles, not formulas, gives independence to the process of wellness and makes more educated consumers of us all.

It's been several years since I wrote the earlier versions of this book. So much new information, experience, feedback, and so many new realizations and scientific advances have driven me to completely rewrite it all and present the information in a more expansive, comprehensive, better-illustrated and more multi-dimensional way.

In addition, the birth of the Primal Body—Primal Mind Web site is an inspiration whose time has come (www.PrimalBody-PrimalMind. com). The field of nutritional science is now evolving exponentially and far faster than ever before. We live in exciting if not perilous times. The Primal Body—Primal Mind web site is an up-to-date and evolving resource for ongoing detailed, cutting edge nutritional information and education. It is for anyone seeking to expand their knowledge, radically improve their health and maximize their mind and its performance to the fullest extent.

Addressing diet from an evolutionary perspective has been of immeasurable value in my practice and seems to speak in a common sense way to even the most hardened skeptic—this includes even avowed junk-food junkies and devout vegetarians or vegans. A respectfully conveyed, common-sense approach, combined with the hard science of basic human physiology, cuts through a lot. Newfound advances in the science of longevity research has added an entirely new dimension to these foundational concepts and promises to radically transform even the healthiest person into manifestations of even greater potential. The implications are truly staggering.

We are boldly venturing here into new and extremely exciting frontiers never before imagined!

My interest is not to prescribe or dictate anyone's dietary habits. The information presented speaks for itself. Ample quality reference material is provided throughout to allow for further exploration. What readers choose to do with the information contained here remains entirely up to them. It has been wisely stated that it is abjectly impossible to actually teach anyone anything. The best one can do is inspire others to learn.

May you find this book inspiring.

Nora T. Gedgaudas, CNS, CNT
Portland, Oregon
August, 2008

For more information relating to neurofeedback, see my web site at www.northwest-neurofeedback.com.

PART ONE:
PRIMAL BODY

*Science is in trouble whenever the will to believe overwhelms
the duty to doubt.*
—Siegfried Othmer, Ph.D.
Chief Scientist, EEG Institute

INTRODUCTION

Just what is it that genuinely constitutes a *healthy diet?*

Innumerable popular books, articles and testimonials overwhelm and confound the average consumer in such a way as to render such a concept virtually meaningless. Misinformation driven by financial interests and emotional biases either sway the gullible to extremes or lead the skeptical-minded to cynicism. Either way, the truth is lost somewhere in the static and remains overwhelmingly clouded. It is my objective in writing this book to put forth an appeal to what can readily be defined as logical and sensible, as well as provide information that is sound from evolutionary, modern scientific and physiological perspectives. This book thinks outside the box of accepted dogma— away from corporate vested interests—and lays a clear foundation of *principles,* rather than *formulas,* that may serve as a guide. This is not just another "caveman" diet book or just another low-carb diet. Fasten your seatbelts.

The optimal human diet is not something that should have to require overly careful formulation by calories or percentages; much less by blood type. One should not require a calorie-counter, a percentages guide or any sort of manual in tow when going to the market to buy food. No one should require a blood test to determine blood-type in order to know how to eat. Such tools, though they provide a seductive sense of structure and/or security, can be unnecessarily confusing and do not ultimately constitute a sound, principle-based, common sense approach. Long term, these approaches tend to lack sustainability.

Fundamentally, as humans, we are much more alike physiologically than not. Although it's true that we need to take into account something called *biochemical individuality,* the fact is that we are all subject to the same fundamental physiological laws. We all share a sophisticated endocrine system subject to certain inter-hormonal relationships; we all, of necessity, have a blood pH ranging between 7.35 and 7.45; and we all have similar basic nutrient requirements. There are certain basic principles that apply to all of us that must be taken into account. To be fair, some of these truths are newly discovered and decidedly alter the landscape of dietary optimization. But there's much more to it than this—much more.

So where do we begin?

All of the structure and functions of the human body are built from and run on nutrients. ALL of them.
—JANET LANG, BA, DC

A LOOK AT WHERE OUR DIETARY REQUIREMENTS ORIGINATED

All humans require similar ranges of both macro and micronutrients and all human groups have similar anatomical, physiological and endocrine functions in regard to diet and nutrition. We were all hunter-gatherers dependent upon wild plants and animals, and these selective pressures shaped our present day nutritional requirements.
—LOREN CORDAIN, PHD, professor of exercise and sports science at Colorado State University and noted evolutionary diet researcher

99.99% of our genes were formed before the development of agriculture.
—DR. S. BOYD EATON, MD, Medical Anthropologist

As a species, we are essentially genetically identical with respect to genetic expression, regardless of blood type, to those humans living more than forty thousand years ago. Our physiologies are fundamentally Paleolithic, which refers to the human evolutionary time period spanning from roughly 2.6 million to about 10 thousand years ago—before the dawn of agriculture. We are the result of an optimal design, shaped and molded by nature over a hundred thousand or so generations. In other words, we are *all*—biologically, genetically and physiologically, without exception—hunter-gatherers. And for much of our hominid evolution, we have been mostly hunters.

The *hunter-gatherer diet* may be defined via at least two different perspectives: Ice-Age Paleolithic, and post-Ice Age, or neo-Paleolithic. The diet of post/neo-Paleolithic peoples, including modern-day hunter-gatherers with some regional variation, essentially consisted of high quality animal source protein, both cooked and uncooked (including organ meats of wild game, all clean) that is hormone-, antibiotic- and pesticide-free, naturally organic, and entirely range-fed with no genetic alterations; some eggs, when available; insects, sorry to say; and/or seafood.

This diet was typically moderately high in fat—which was highly coveted—estimated to have been at roughly ten times our modern intake. This included varieties of saturated forms, monounsaturated, omega-3, and balanced quantities of omega-6, together with abundant fat-soluble nutrients. Post-Ice Age primitive human diets, as well as diets during more temperate periods amidst the Ice Age, generally included a significant variety of vegetable matter, some fresh raw nuts and seeds, and some very limited quantities of tart, wild fruit, as was seasonally available.

There was far more plant material in the diets of our more recent ancestors than our more ancient hominid ancestors, due to different factors. We have spent 90–95% of the last 500,000 years locked in the grip of mostly ice and snow via the Ice Age, with only the briefest cool periods of reprieve, when edible plant life might have grown over a significant portion of this planet. Even while the Northern Hemisphere was gripped in snow and ice, Africa was being ripped apart by drought and wildfires. Studies of ancient human *coprolites,* or fossilized human feces dating anywhere from 300,000 to as recent as 50,000 years ago, have revealed essentially a complete lack of any plant material in the human diets of the subjects studied. In other words, it is likely we subsisted for a very significant portion of our evolution almost solely upon the meat and fat of animals we hunted. Fat was *the* prime commodity for its concentrated nutrient and energy value. As omnivores and opportunists, we would have certainly procured whatever might have been available to us for food. Permafrost and drought, however, left limited options.

Another important limitation stems from the fact that we as a species have only relatively recently developed a universally controlled use of fire. By most accounts, this did not occur before 50,000 to 100,000 years ago. Although scattered evidence of fire exists from as far back as 300,000 to 400,000 years ago, it is unlikely that sophisticated development of cooking practices occurred much before the use of fire became more universal and commonplace—sometime after Cro-Magnon man migrated into Europe. (The oldest known pottery dates only as far back as 6800 BC, incidentally.)

What makes the use of cooking especially significant relates to the toxicity of most plant species. Wild plants contain any number of toxic compounds that would have made their use as food in any significant quantity perilous. Cooking is the only means by which many of these anti-nutrients can be neutralized. Modern produce has been genetically modified to reduce the presence of harmful compounds to a significant extent.

Most wild plants, on the other hand, require extremely careful selection and preparation. Most starchy roots, tubers and legumes would have been prohibitively dangerous to consume without extensive cooking. Furthermore, the energy expended in the procurement of remaining types of plant foods easily exceeds their potential caloric value, to say little of their meager, inferior available protein content so critical to our needs. Mass die-off of mega-fauna following the last Ice Age 10,000 years ago and over-hunting by humans probably lead to an increased dependence upon plant foods, and ultimately to the development of agriculture. Nonetheless, it is widely postulated that it was, in fact, our extended dependence on the meat and fat of animals (rich in eicosapentaenoic acid, or EPA; and docosahexaenoic acid, or DHA) through these frozen winters of unimaginable duration that allowed for the rapid enlargement and development of the human brain.

Our increased dependence on hunting also likely helped facilitate and develop the very qualities human qualities that we most intrinsically value—cunning, cooperation, altruism, sharing, advanced creativity, the power to foresee, to be able call upon the past in terms of the future, the capacity to evaluate with complexity, to imagine solutions—qualities not particularly found in other primates. Also, interestingly, the dominant form of fatty acids in the human brain is omega-3; in chimps and other primates, it is mostly omega-6—a very significant distinction, and one that is the likely result of these Ice Age dietary changes.

Many authors popularizing the notion of Paleolithic diets base their conclusive evidence on the diets of more contemporary primitive peoples, forgetting that for most of our evolution, the world has been a very, very different place. Either way, it is evident from even the most recent analysis of primitive diets that animal-source foods and fat-soluble nutrients invariably play a critical, central role in extraordinary physical and mental health and freedom from disease. It is also quite evident that diets consisting of any significant quantity of carbohydrates are a strictly modern phenomenon, one that our Ice Age human physiology has evolved little adaptation to, or defense against.

Carbohydrates, other than the largely indigestible variety found in fibrous vegetables and greens, have generally played a minimal role at best through most of human evolution. Fruit was only consumed seasonally by our post-Ice Age ancestors in most places; wild fruit is extremely fibrous and isn't that sweet. Many potatoes and tubers would have required extensive cooking to neutralize extremely toxic alkaloids. Wild varieties that would have been available to us through most of our history as a species can be especially toxic.

In other words, it isn't likely we were eating baked potatoes with our wooly mammoth steaks—or much starch at all.

In fact, of all the macro-nutrients (that is, protein, fats and carbohydrates), the only one for which there is *no* actual human dietary requirement is carbohydrates. This is a critical and very fundamental point to remember.

Our bodies can manufacture glucose, as needed, from a combination of protein and fat in the diet. As a matter of fact, glucose is really only needed for fueling our red blood cells. Most tissues in the body, including the brain, actually prefer, if we let them, to use *ketones,* the energy-producing by-product from the metabolism of fats. This fact is very overlooked by the majority of medical and nutritional experts. There is abundant evidence that many modern disease processes, including cardiovascular disease, elevated triglycerides, obesity, hypertension, diabetes, hypoglycemia and cancer, to name a few, are the product *not* of excess natural fat in the diet, but of excess carbohydrates. Other contributing factors certainly include ultra-prevalent unnatural trans fats, rancid fats, unnaturally high quantities of dietary omega-6 fatty acids from vegetable oils, heavy metals and other pollutants, artificial chemicals and additives and widespread use of xenoestrogens, the artificial estrogen-like compounds used in pesticides, plastics and many other common household items and cleaning supplies.

Current marketing ploys and diet dictocrats unrelentingly cling to other notions, in spite of overwhelming and well-documented evidence to the contrary. More modern ills can be traced to chronic carbohydrate consumption than any other single factor. Trans fats might come in at a close second.

Consider, for instance, that the first four cases of coronary thrombosis ever recorded were written up in the *Journal of the American Medical Association* in 1912. This disease was unknown by the medical profession before that time, and it was considered an unusual disorder. Dr. Paul Dudley White, personal physician to President Eisenhower and author of the very first medical textbook on coronary heart disease, had never heard the words "coronary thrombosis" when he graduated medical school in 1911. When, as a physician, he decided to specialize in this newly emerging field of "coronary heart disease," his colleagues suggested he find an area of specialty that was more profitable. By the 1950s, it was among the leading causes of death among Americans. However, the consumption of animal proteins and saturated fat had been going on for a hundred thousand generations prior to that time. What had suddenly changed?

The quality, nutrient-rich dietary fats richly present in the organ meats, fatty fish, bone marrow and tallows favored by humans throughout 2.6 million years of evolution, constituted 60% *or more* of some contemporary primitive cultures' caloric intake—all without detriment to the heart. This consumption of naturally occurring dietary fat did not, all of a sudden, become problematic. It was, in fact, the advent of the food industry, leading to increased consumption of refined "Franken-foods," vegetable or hydrogenated trans fats, and sugar or carbohydrates, which more clearly correlate to such statistics.

And it was the combined egos of medical theoreticians and the greedy, unscrupulous design of members of the vegetable oil industry that gave birth to and perpetuated the myth of the dietary heart hypothesis. The dietary heart hypothesis sought to vilify saturated fat and cholesterol as the culprits in heart disease. What started out as a plausible hypothesis has never, *ever* been proven, despite extensive effort and millions of dollars spent. Today there are literally billions upon billions of dollars—spanning from government agencies, medical establishment interests, the pharmaceutical industry, organizations such as the American Heart Association and, let's not forget, the ever-popular food industry—all invested in the perpetuation of the anti-saturated fat and anti-cholesterol agenda. This sordid history is well-documented, though poorly publicized, as the media is beholding to its corporate advertisers.

As noted by Dr. George V. Mann, noted researcher in the Framingham Heart Study: ". . . on-going issues of pride, profit and prejudice cause outdated and never-proven notions of the saturated fat/cholesterol hypotheses to persist despite a lack of supportive evidence in the medical literature."

USDA data from the early 1900s clearly shows a dramatic shifts away from animal fats and increases in the consumption of industrially produced vegetable oils, hydrogenated or trans fats like margarine or Crisco, refined flours and, of course, sugar.

Note the following illustrations:

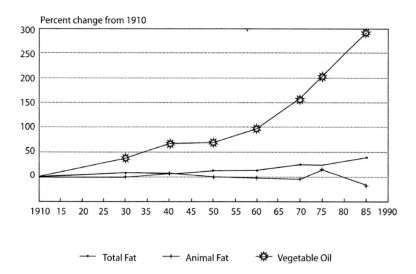

Source of data: USDA
Changes in per capita availablity of dietary fats in the United States.

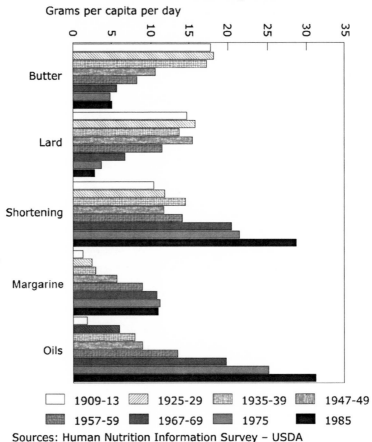

U.S. Dietary Fats
Table and Cooking Sources

Grams per capita per day

Butter

Lard

Shortening

Margarine

Oils

☐ 1909-13   ▨ 1925-29   ▦ 1935-39   ▨ 1947-49
▦ 1957-59   ■ 1967-69   ▦ 1975   ■ 1985

Sources: Human Nutrition Information Survey – USDA

Enter: the Food Industry.

It is increasingly clear from current medical literature that much chronic, degenerative and other uniquely modern disease processes are readily attributable not to natural saturated fats and cholesterol but to something increasingly known as *syndrome X,* more recently referred to as *metabolic syndrome.* Essentially, insulin-resistance. Syndrome X or metabolic syndrome is both created and exacerbated by primarily chronic carbohydrate consumption, in combination with dietary trans fats, unnaturally abundant omega-6 (vegetable oils) and, to some extent, possibly even excess omega-9 (oleic and olive oils).

Other contributors to insulin resistance include: stress, food sensitivities, dieting, caffeine and other stimulants, sleep deprivation, alcohol, tobacco, steroids, lack of exercise, all prescription or over-the-counter and/or recreational drugs, and excess or unnecessary thyroid replacement therapy. *Most importantly, insulin resistance is primarily a phenomenon associated with a diet deficient in protein and fats while consuming excess carbohydrates.* (Diane Schwarzbein, 1999)

It seems reasonable to suggest that resistance to insulin-mediated glucose disposal and the manner in which the organism responds to this defect play major roles in the pathogenesis and clinical course of what are often referred to as diseases of Western civilization.
—GERALD M. REAVEN, MD, 1995

It is clear that low-fat diets, promoted by numerous U.S. government agencies and even more numerous heavily funded health organizations have not prevented: heart disease (which is still on the rise); obesity (now affecting more than an estimated 58% of the American public); diabetes (the most common end-result of insulin resistance— now recognized by the World Health Organization as epidemic, affecting as many as three out of five persons and rapidly rising, even in children); cancer (now exceeding heart disease as the leading cause of death in the United States); or any of the other disease processes low (saturated)-fat eating is supposed to prevent. The numbers continue to climb.

Mood disorders, learning disabilities, ADD/HD, autism, Asperger's syndrome, anxiety disorders and immune or auto-immune related diseases are also equally unprecedented in our history and are rapidly on the rise. Although total dietary fat consumption has risen since 1900, fats coming from animal sources have substantially decreased in the American diet, while dietary vegetable fats, including trans fats, have risen almost exponentially. And many of these fats have entered the human diet for the first time in human evolution within the last hundred years. In fact, the number one source fat calories in America today comes from soybean oil, nearly all of which is partially hydrogenated and a prevalent source of dangerous trans fat.

Concomitantly, the percentage of the Western diet comprised of carbohydrates, from all sources, is of a proportion equally unprecedented in all of human history. The overall, number-one source of dietary calories at this time in the United States is actually *high fructose corn syrup,* an extremely toxic industrial sweetener found in nearly all processed foods.

The diet-heart hypothesis (that suggests that high intake of fat and cholesterol causes heart disease) has been repeatedly shown to be wrong, and yet, for complicated reasons of pride, profit and prejudice, the hypothesis continues to be exploited by scientists, fund-raising enterprises, food companies, and even governmental agencies. The public is being deceived by the greatest health scam of the century.
—GEORGE V. MANN, MD, formerly with the Framingham Project

The agricultural revolution did not take place until five to ten thousand years ago, probably as a result of necessity, with increasing human populations and a decreased availability of wild game in certain regions of the world. This may have been due in part to extinctions of mega-fauna following the last Ice Age, and possibly over-hunting. Implementation of agriculture was far from an immediately universal phenomenon, however, and thousands of hunter-gatherer societies continued to thrive worldwide. Recent estimation asserts that agriculture was not widely implemented in Europe until little more than 2,000 years ago. By most accounts, it takes roughly 40,000–100,000 years for human genetic expression to adapt significantly to such major changes.

Consequently, it is logical to conclude and easy to demonstrate that modern agricultural foods such as grains and legumes, corn, wheat, soy, etc., are foods that are *not* especially compatible—particularly when consumed in any significant quantity—with optimal human health. Grain consumption has been linked with allergies, food sensitivities, auto-immune disorders, colon cancer, pancreatic disorders, mineral deficiencies, celiac disease, epilepsy, cerebellar ataxias, dementia, degenerative brain/central nervous system diseases, peripheral neuropathies, of axonal or demyelinating type, and myopathies, as well as autism and schizophrenia, to name a few (Cordain, 2002).

There was, in fact, a marked decline in human stature, bone density, dental development and health, including an increase in birth defects, malnutrition and degenerative disease, following the early implementation of agricultural lifestyle. Anthropologists and archaeologists know this well. Legumes, too, are particularly rich in starch—roughly 60% of their composition—and contain numerous anti-nutrients that can cause mineral deficiencies and other problems.

Our more modern ability to transport fresh produce and broader varieties of fresh foods during all seasons throughout much of the industrialized world allows for greater varieties of foods in various regions and has helped improve health considerably. Such advances, unfortunately, are entirely dependent on the use of limited fossil fuels. Even those cultures adopting the early agricultural lifestyle typically included as many animal source foods as were available to them.

No known primitive culture in the history of the human species has ever adopted vegetarianism by choice.

It is a popular misconception that prehistoric humans usually died when they were around twenty years old, so it didn't matter how much meat, fat or how few carbohydrates they ate, because they didn't live long enough to develop heart disease or any of the other modern disorders that meat and fat consumption supposedly cause. This twenty- to forty-year figure that is commonly batted around as the average age of death for prehistoric humans is no more than exactly that: the *average* age of death. It incorporates infant mortality as well. The figure, often misrepresented, states nothing about the rate of aging or maximum lifespan of our prehistoric ancestors. "Other methods of determining true probable lifespan, as well as a look at modern hunter-gatherer societies, show it was probably about the same as ours" (Eades, 2000).

It is important to also note that the above figures are frequently confused with post-agricultural time period mortality statistics.

It is clear that post-agricultural peoples became shorter in stature, had much higher rates of osteoporosis, rickets and other bone mineral disorders. They were also plagued with vitamin and mineral deficiencies not shared by their stone-age ancestors: scurvy, beriberi, pellagra, vitamin A and zinc deficiencies, together with iron deficiency anemia—all endemic to cereal-based diets. They suffered tooth decay, skeletal abnormalities and mal-occluded dental arches. They had infectious diseases in far greater numbers, more childhood mortality and decidedly shorter life spans. Prehistoric or pre-agricultural humans had the capability to live as long as we do without all our high-tech " healthcare"; they simply didn't have as comparatively controlled an environment, and as a result, were far more prone to accident and infection. In other words, "what we're actually comparing when we compare our average age of death to theirs is, in reality, the relative hostility of our two environments" (Eades, 2000).

This is also misleading, however, since it is clear that primitive societies did not suffer the same ranges of degenerative or chronic disease shared by their early agricultural descendants or among our modern-day populace. Primary causes of death in stone-age societies were typically accident and infection. If one managed to get around those two primary causes of death, as well as infant mortality, one stood a good chance of leading a long, healthful and vibrant life, free of most of the chronic and degenerative diseases so prevalent in our aging populations today.

It is also a popular misconception that primitive cultures were a great deal more physically active than modern humans are today and could therefore afford to eat a diet higher in fat and calories. The evidence from numerous anthropological studies of hunter-gatherer cultures suggest a typical "work-day" of no more than about three hours, including procurement of food, housing and clothing. And there were no jogging shoes or gym memberships. This is in sharp contrast to the lifestyle of post-agricultural farmers known to work eight or more hours a day performing often-backbreaking labor in the field. Agriculture may have spawned civilization (not to mention over-population), but it clearly was not the fast track to easy living or radiant health. We paid a price for the change, as has our beleaguered planetary environment.

The bottom line is that we achieved most, if not all, our dietary or physiological requirements long before the agricultural revolution and those requirements have not changed.

Diets consistent with these principles and a substantially higher nutrient intake, particularly of the fat-soluble nutrients, according to numerous anthropological studies, have, for hundreds of thousands of years, been consistent with superior health, strong lean physical structure and freedom from chronic or degenerative illnesses so common today.

And high carbohydrate consumption, sugary, starchy and/or refined—and the vast tidal waves of insulin generated as a result—are
a strictly modern phenomenon our primitive physiologies are ill-suited for. One only need go and stand at a Safeway checkout line to see
what the majority of people place on the checkout conveyer belt; and
one can visibly see how that has affected their physical, and even mental, health. It certainly stands to reason that if something on the grocery store shelf would not have looked like food to someone walking
around with a loin cloth and a spear forty or fifty thousand years ago,
it probably isn't food for us now, either. (See the following Average
Contemporary Hunter-Gatherer Nutrient Intake table.)

Average Contemporary Hunter-Gatherer Nutrient Intake*

Nutrient	Paleolithic Intake	RDA	U.S. Intake
Vitamin C	604 mg	60 mg	77–109 mg
Vitamin E	33 mg	8–10 mg	7–10 mg
Calcium	1,956 mg	800–1200 mg	750 mg
Magnesium	700 mg	350 mg	250 mg
Potassium	10,500 mg	3,500 mg	2,500 mg
Zinc	43 mg	12–15 mg	5–14 mg
Fiber	50–104 grams	25–35 grams	10 grams

*(Eaton, SB, Eaton SB III, Konner MJ. Paleolithic nutrition revisited: twelve
year retrospective on its nature and implications. *European Journal of Clinical
Nutrition* 1997); 51: 207–216

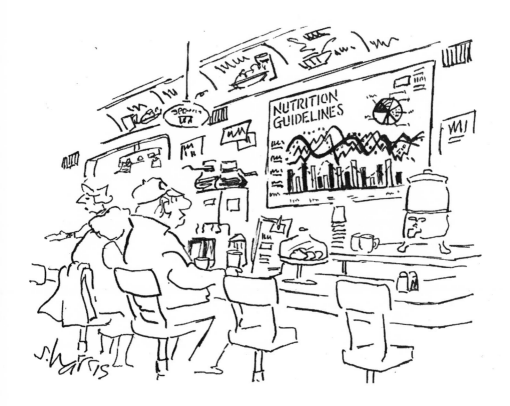

THE PREHISTORIC FOOD PYRAMID THE USDA (AND OTHER VESTED INTERESTS) DIDN'T WANT YOU TO SEE

If one were to construct a food pyramid designed around a diet close-ly resembling that of our pre-agricultural ancestors, it would most eas-ily appear as the following—mercifully leaving out insects and grubs, for the sake of more delicate modern-day culinary sensibilities:

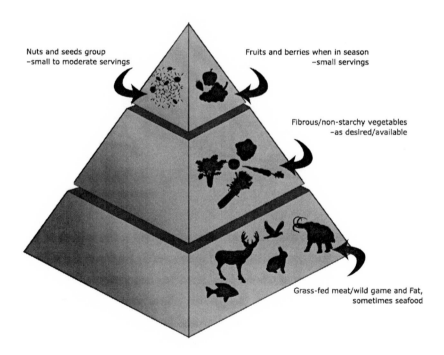

Nuts and seeds group
–small to moderate servings

Fruits and berries when in season
–small servings

Fibrous/non-starchy vegetables
–as desired/available

Grass-fed meat/wild game and Fat,
sometimes seafood

This clearly contrasts with the largely scientifically unfounded USDA Food Pyramid so commonly promoted by registered dietitians and nutritionists, the same people who design hospital food and school lunches.

No human society in history has consumed a diet remotely resembling what the USDA Pyramid suggests as optimal.

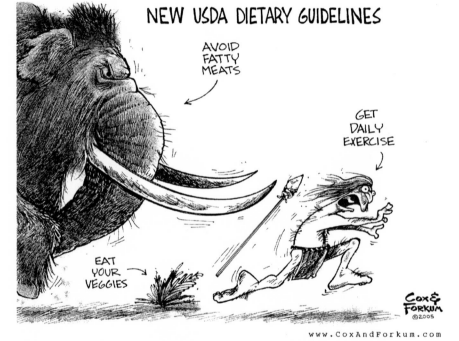

www.CoxAndForkum.com

There are more than fifteen thousand papers on the subject of Paleolithic or primitive nutrition, and innumerable books on the subject written by a variety of scholars and scientists in a variety of fields. No one owns this information, though many have borrowed from it. This is not a formulary approach to diet and health that requires a written guide. It is not a fad diet—or if it is, then it's the oldest fad diet known to humankind. Eating a diet as similar as possible to what our ancestors ate is purely common sense and based entirely on how we have been genetically molded for the vast majority of human evolution. No gurus needed. Eat the way your body was designed for you to eat, and a lot takes care of itself.

The USDA Food Pyramid should be renamed "The Feedlot Pyramid." It's nutrient profile is the same as swine fattening chow. And it is fattening the population in the same way.
—DRS. MICHAEL AND MARY DAN EADES, MD, 2000

ARE GENES REALLY EVERYTHING THEY'RE CRACKED UP TO BE?

A great deal of press is being given today to the idea that we may have—through no fault of our own—a silent killer, or two or three, lurking in the entanglement of DNA deep within our cells. It's the ultimate boogeyman: a terrorist "sleeper cell" right inside our own bodies, lying in wait for just the right moment to unleash its deadliest intent. Everyone is running to get tested for their genetic profiles in an effort to prepare for the unspeakable inevitability of any number of diseases. The medical establishment, not unlike homeland security, could not be more delighted to feed the rampant paranoia and offer, at a price, everything from pharmaceutical to surgical preventatives to help save us from ourselves.

Although there is certainly some merit to the science of genetics, its revelations are more commonly abused, or blown entirely out of proportion, than related to any actual threat. Our genes really aren't that special. We all have twenty-two thousand of them, far fewer than the Human Genome Project expected to find. We all have all sorts of genes for all sorts of things, good and bad. Not all are actively expressed—a decidedly good thing. Many remain dormant. Genes, however, do not switch on and off randomly, like the randomly spun, bullet-containing cartridge in a gun, playing Russian roulette. *A gene will not express itself at all unless the environment surrounding it becomes favorable to that expression.* A cancer gene, for instance, needs certain environmental requirements to be met before it can activate. In other words:

It's the environment, stupid!
—BRUCE LIPTON, PHD, 2005

Even by the most conservative standards in genetics, we actually control anywhere from a "low" of 80% to upwards of 97% or more of our own genetic expression with respect to potential disease processes, and even longevity. Genes are turned on and off by regulatory genes, and *regulatory genes are controlled mainly by nutrients.* The thing to consider here is that our genes reside within the cells and the nutrients that best protect them from mutation or undesirable influences are those which are best able to cross the cellular membrane into the matrix of the cell. For this, *fat-soluble* nutrients and antioxidants are critical . . . and long overlooked and underestimated in importance and value.

Those with vested interests in keeping you hostage to the illusion of your own inner "genetic threat" would rather you weren't aware of the fact that there is *no drug* anywhere that can regulate genetic expression better or more powerfully than diet.

SO, WHAT'S FOR DINNER?

Although it is nearly impossible to replicate a truly Paleolithic diet in our modern everyday life (who has time to hunt and gather any more?), certain fundamental principles are easily derived and applied.

It is important to emphasize that once upon a time, literally everything we ate was both free-range, fully grass fed and organic. It should be obvious that factory-farmed, chemically, hormonally antibiotic and pesticide-laden meat, further insulted by irradiation to extend shelf life, is not quality food. Such animals also lead tortured lives, fed foods that are unnatural to them, including grain, which is used to fatten them up (take a hint). Grain-fattened animals yield a distinctly altered fatty-acid profile with unnaturally high omega-6 levels and virtually no omega-3, which is otherwise found in highly significant quantities in wild game and exclusively pasture-fed animals. The same is true, unfortunately, of farm-raised seafood (see the following illustration, borrowed with permission from Jo Robinson's book, *Pasture Perfect,* 2000). It is also

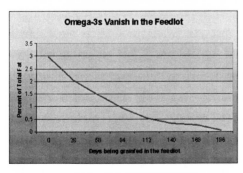

Data from: J Animal Sci (1993) 71(8):2079-88.

logical to conclude that genetically engineered, pesticide-laden produce grown in mineral-depleted soils do not promote optimal health or longevity.

This being said, it can be a comfort to know that it is entirely possible to obtain clean, quality, humanely raised grass-fed poultry and eggs, beef, lamb and organ meats. These can come from easily available sources ranging from various co-ops, certain grocery markets, as well as directly from the farmers themselves. For the more adventuresome, venison, elk, buffalo, ostrich and other more exotic varieties of game meat may be found via the Internet and some of the better meat counters (although these can be expensive). Wild-caught seafood of all kinds, organic vegetables and greens, seeds, fresh nuts, berries and some (just some) fruit are abundantly available.

Eating never has to be dull. Nor need it be too costly.

Some may argue that this seems like it would be an expensive way to eat. Putting aside the alternative specter of the eventual and ongoing health costs associated with the modern, conventional Western diet, one can save a tremendous amount of revenue merely avoiding processed, pre-packaged, refined, nutrient-devoid junk foods and beverages—and put the savings from that toward whole, unprocessed organic vegetables and free-range meats with a minimum of financial difficulty. Nutrient-dense quality meats, fats and vegetables are readily satisfying, and smaller amounts of food are far more filling. Naturally occurring fat, which our ancestors would have sought out as much as possible, is inherently satisfying to the appetite.

It is also a simple matter in many places to either grow a small vegetable garden in one's own in backyard or community-garden plot or shop seasonal farmers' markets, where produce is most affordable. Community Supported Agriculture (CSA) programs are abundant and allow for considerable savings on a huge variety of organic, bio-dynamically grown produce—especially when orders are split with friends or neighbors. And organic, free range, exclusively grass-fed meat, poultry, and eggs, even raw milk can be readily purchased from family farms in your area. This is highly recommended, as one can readily purchase meats in larger quantities to be stored in a chest-freezer for convenience and considerable long-term savings.

This is also an advantage from the standpoint of having firsthand knowledge of where one's food is actually coming from—something conspicuously lacking in our modern-day world. Personally, I would much rather support the honest and ethical efforts of a small local family farmer, than the vast faceless and greed-driven food industry or the conglomerates of factory farms who care nothing for the nutritional content of what they produce, the health of their consumers or the environment. For others, hunting or fishing for their food can be a viable option. This does not have to be expensive! Good quality food can be within almost anyone's financial reach with a little resourcefulness and, initially, at least, a little extra time.

Contacting a local chapter of the Weston A. Price Foundation can put one in touch with resources, recipes, cooking classes and other families with which one can seek support and helpful ideas. Members may pool resources together to purchase CSAs and can be a wealth of information. See www.WestonAPrice.org for details. Additional resources for locating grass-fed meats, etc., as well as other useful Web sites, may be found in Appendix-E of this book. A summary of general guidelines and suggestions for getting started on your road to health is in Appendix-A.

Things to generally avoid, aside from the obvious

Excess consumption of sugar, starch and cereal-based carbohydrates *is easily the most destructive dietary tendency today*. It is a rampant problem leading to heart disease, obesity, diabetes, cancer and many other degenerative disorders, as well as numerous mental health and cognitive problems.

As a whole, it is entirely preferable to avoid starch—such as that found in rice and white or red potatoes, which contain easily a quarter cup or more of very high glycemic, glycating sugar—as well as cereals, breads, pastas and conventionally produced dairy.

Milk, especially the "low-fat" variety, is very high in carbohydrates; heavy cream, however, has essentially none. Some traditional societies who raised grass-fed sheep, goats and cattle were shown to thrive on raw, whole fat, unpasteurized and organic, grass-fed (hormone-, antibiotic- and pesticide-free), un-homogenized milk, cream, cheese and nutrient-rich butter. Such dairy sources are commercially unavailable at this time in most public markets, with the exception of some imported raw milk cheeses (Delicious!) and online quality raw dairy sources (see www.organicpastures.com). Some states in which certified raw milk products are legal can be found by contacting A Campaign for Real Milk (www.RealMilk.org), or via www.eatwild. com. (Nationwide sources of grass-fed meats may also be found on this Web site.)

Small amounts of raw, unprocessed dairy products can be healthful, if desired, and well tolerated. Butter and heavy cream can be used more liberally.

Pasteurized and especially *ultra*-pasteurized milk products contain rancid fats and oxidized cholesterol. There is also a theory that homogenization may render a natural component in milk fat, *xanthine oxidase,* a particularly dangerous substance that some scientists believe may possibly produce atherosclerotic lesions by breaking down plasmalogen, the cellular "glue" holding arterial cells together, in human arterial walls. It is possible to find organic whole milk products that are un-homogenized in many natural foods-type markets. Low fat (skim, 1% and 2%) milks contain large amounts of oxidized cholesterol: powdered, denatured whole milk gets added in after the cream is removed in processing to add "body" to the texture. These milk products are made up mainly of carbohydrates and should be entirely avoided.

Raw, organic, pasture-fed butter can be an especially rich source of commonly deficient and beneficial nutrients, including vitamin A, conjugated linolenic acid (CLA) and selenium, as well as a beneficial substance known as *X-factor,* found only in entirely pasture-fed butter. In addition, raw butter, milk and cream contain the Wulzen factor, otherwise known as the "anti-stiffness" factor, beneficial for healthy joints. Butter, a wonderful source of true vitamin A and selenium, can be healthfully included more liberally in the diet.

Fast foods and processed snack foods like chips, crackers and rice cakes should *always* be avoided—they are laden with dangerous trans fats, or processed and/or rancid fats, excess carbohydrates, chemical additives and carcinogens. Save your hard-earned money for real food.

GRAINS . . . ARE THEY REALLY
A HEALTH FOOD?

Grains and legumes typically contain very high levels of a substance known as *phytic acid*. Phytic acid actively binds minerals and eliminates them from the body and results, with increased consumption, in widespread mineral deficiencies, including calcium, iron, magnesium and zinc. Legumes typically containing 60% starch and only relatively small amounts of *incomplete* protein, also contain potent protease inhibitors, which can damage one's ability to properly digest and utilize dietary protein, as well as damage the pancreas over time, when over-depended upon as a source of calories.

Careful preparation by pre-soaking, sprouting or fermenting these foods can minimize or even eliminate phytic acid and other anti-nutrients. *Nonetheless, they remain a very high carbohydrate food source.* If these foods are desired (preferably in minimal amounts) and are tolerated, it is always best to treat them by such methods first. It is important to be aware, however, that phytic acid and trypsin inhibitors in soybeans can only be neutralized by means of fermentation. The excellent and educational book and cookbook *Nourishing Traditions,* by Sally Fallon, details such food preparation methods and is filled with accurate, fascinating nutritional information and marvelous recipes. The book is based more in traditional-type diets, rather than specifically Paleolithic culinary approaches, however.

Grains and legumes also contain goitrogens, or thyroid-inhibiting substances, as well as "foreign proteins" like gluten, and are an extremely common source of allergies and sensitivities that can lead to both physical and mental or emotional disorders, even when the best preparation methods are used. One additional hypothesis suggests that the lack of essential amino acid L-tryptophan in grains, now an unnatural and primary food source for commercially raised beef and poultry (not to mention humans), may help account for rampant serotonin deficiencies, clinical depression, anxiety and some forms of ADD in our populations. Carbohydrate consumption, in general, depletes serotonin stores, as well as greatly depletes the B-vitamins needed to convert amino acids to many needed neurotransmitters.

As there is *no human dietary grain requirement*—and since grain consumption causes so many known health problems due to its anti-nutrient content, its tryptophan-poor profile, high omega-6 levels, and its mainly starch-based content, as well as its allergy and sensitivity potential—there is *little reason to include grains in the diet of anyone seeking optimal health.*

In fact, the fewer grains consumed the better. Zero is by far best.

The Weston A. Price Foundation, with whom I am proudly affiliated by membership, maintains that grains are okay, since many more traditional post-agricultural societies were seemingly able to incorporate them healthfully as long as they are properly prepared (that is, pre-soaked, fermented and/or sprouted). But rapid changes in the genetic robustness of our species, in our culture, particularly, and especially poor prenatal diets over the last generation or two have rendered many in today's world—particularly our children—more vulnerable and much more intolerant of grains, legumes, starch, milk, sugar, especially, and other post-agricultural and processed foods in any form. These are also very high-carbohydrate foods.

Our genetic resilience has changed and is continuing to change for the worse at an alarming rate. Health in this country is declining rapidly; many degenerative processes and illnesses once thought to affect only our aging population are now afflicting the young . . . and sometimes the very young.

The money spent today in the United States on medical interventions for every imaginable type of illness is staggering. We are number one in the world in medical spending. By the year 2016, what Americans spend on so-called " healthcare"—already an astronomical *$2 trillion*—is expected to *double* to more than *$4 trillion,* according to economists with the National Health Statistics Group. Already, *sixteen cents out of every American dollar is spent on healthcare.* This will rise to nearly twenty cents in ten years. Consequently, out-of-pocket consumer spending on healthcare will rise to *$440 billion.* Things are going, from bad to worse, fast.

It is currently estimated (conservatively) that one in every 200 people suffers from celiac disease, a devastating consequence of gluten consumption for some. Some hypothesize that this number may be closer to one in 30. Gluten containing grains include wheat (e.g., durum, graham, semolina, kamut, spelt, as well as rye, barley, oats and triticale). Many, if not most, who suffer from this condition do so completely unaware of the dangerous vulnerability within themselves.

Although a biopsy of the small intestine is commonly used to diagnose celiac disease, fully six out of ten celiac sufferers exhibit no intestinal or GI symptoms at all. Although there are numerous methods for assessing gluten sensitivity, most are somewhat unreliable in their accuracy. I've found that a more accurate assessment may be made by using a stool antibody test from EnteroLab (www.enterolab.com). Their Web site also contains extremely helpful information on the subject and includes accurate testing for other common food sensitivities as well.

Brain and mood disorders, osteoporosis, diabetes, cardiovascular diseases, bowel diseases, autoimmune diseases, inflammatory disorders and cancer are rampant. Grains are rarely suspected as the original culprit, though every one of these disorders can potentially be traced to an often-insidious gluten intolerance. Gluten sensitivity is only rarely obvious to the afflicted, and many are even surprised to learn they have this sensitivity.

Even though other grains, such as quinoa, millet and buckwheat do not contain gluten, they are still more a source of starch than of protein. Gluten and carbohydrate intolerance, in general, are far more the rule than the exception in today's world. It is logical to conclude that grain consumption, especially gluten-containing grains, just isn't worth the dietary risk, given our culture's innumerable health challenges and vulnerabilities. Why play Russian roulette? Why add to the unnecessary, glycating, fattening and neurotransmitter and hormonally dysregulating carbohydrate load?

It stands to further reason that the more symptoms a person has physically, cognitively or psychologically, the more *primitive,* with respect to dietary choices, one ought to consider going for reclaiming rightful health. The commonality of degenerative diseases does not make these diseases a normal part of aging, or even remotely inevitable.

The choice is mostly ours.

DON'T GET GREASED BY VEGETABLE OILS

Vegetable oils, particularly commercial soybean, safflower, sunflower, corn, cottonseed and canola oils, are an unnatural, very recent addition to the human diet. They are extremely prone to rancidity and cause mutagenic or atherogenic changes in the human body. High consumptions of these oils contribute to premature aging, wrinkles, cancers and many inflammatory processes. They should never, *ever* be used in cooking.

Small amounts of extra-virgin olive oil in salads and a dash or two of sesame oil, which contains a potent heat-protective antioxidant, *sesamin,* for flavoring in medium-heat cooking are fine. Even excess amounts of olive oil, however, along with other vegetable oils, have been shown to interfere with utilization of omega-3 in the diet and have also been shown to enhance insulin resistance (Enig 2002). Omega-3s (in the form of EPA/DHA), in contrast, abundant in wild-caught fish, wild game and exclusively pasture-fed meats, are known to significantly improve insulin sensitivity. Saturated fats like coconut oil, palm oil, butter, lard and tallow are essentially neutral and benign in moderate quantities, some having numerous beneficial antimicrobial properties. They are also important for the proper utilization of both essential fats (omega-3 and 6) and protein in the body.

Margarine, hydrogenated/partially hydrogenated vegetable oils, and vegetable shortenings should be avoided at all costs—these artificial, "plastic" trans fats have no place in human health!

Use a little olive oil on your salads, accent stir-frys with sesame oil, use raw, organic butter liberally on steamed veggies, as it assists in the absorption of oil-soluble nutrients in them. Use coconut oil, organic lard or quality tallow for higher heat cooking or sautéing. These fats are highly stable and will not easily go rancid—and rancid fats are extremely damaging to your body and DNA. Short- and medium-chain saturated fats that are found in butter and coconut oil are far more likely to be used by your body, including the heart and other organs, as energy, rather than stored as body fat.

> **Carbohydrates and unnatural fats—not healthy, natural fats in the diet—make you fat.**

SO WHAT ABOUT SOY?

Contrary to popular belief, soy (particularly tofu, soy milk and soy protein isolate) is among the newest additions to the human diet. Soy has been considered unfit for human consumption since ancient times, but chemical processing methods created by corporate interests have created an "all new" soy, purported to be the cornerstone of health and longevity. The unsuspecting public has unfortunately succumbed to misleading claims and other marketing ploys to increasingly seek out meat substitutes—including texturized vegetable protein (TVP), tofu, soy milk and soy protein powders. Many have been led to believe that these foods somehow prevent cancer and heart disease, and provide improved quality protein in their diets.

Nothing could be further from the truth.

Publicized studies attempting to show health benefits of soy are largely funded and promoted to the media and health food industry by the multi-billion dollar multi-national soy industry in an effort to market their product. Innumerable independent studies, however, suggest considerable reason for concern.

The following is cited from the Weston A. Price Foundation Web site:

- ▸ High levels of phytic acid in soy reduce assimilation of calcium, magnesium, copper, iron and zinc. Phytic acid in soy is *not* neutralized by ordinary preparation methods such as soaking, sprouting and long, slow cooking. High phytate diets have caused growth problems in children. (Also, soy contains the *highest levels* of phytic acid of any grain or legume)

▸ Trypsin inhibitors in soy interfere with protein digestion and may cause pancreatic disorders. In test animals, soy containing trypsin inhibitors caused stunted growth

▸ Soy phytoestrogens disrupt endocrine function and have the potential to cause infertility and to promote breast cancer in adult women

▸ Soy phytoestrogens are potent antithyroid agents (goitrogens) that cause hypothyroidism and may cause thyroid cancer. In infants, consumption of soy formula has been linked to autoimmune thyroid disease

▸ Vitamin B12 analogs in soy are not absorbed and actually increase the body's requirement for vitamin B12

▸ Soy foods increase the body's requirement for vitamin D

▸ Fragile proteins are denatured during high temperature processing to make soy protein isolate and texturized vegetable protein

▸ Processing of soy protein results in the formation of toxic lysinoalanine and highly carcinogenic nitrosamines

▸ Free glutamic acid, or MSG, a potent neurotoxin, is formed during soy food processing and additional amounts are added to many soy foods

▸ Soy foods contain high levels of aluminum, which is toxic to the nervous system and kidneys

▸ Recent studies suggest a link between soy consumption and kidney stones.

Additional concerns (as if all that wasn't bad enough):

Soy has never been given the Generally Recognized as Safe status (GRAS) by the FDA.

Soy is a phyto-endocrine disrupter, inhibiting the thyroid enzyme, thyroid peroxidase, necessary for the synthesis of the hormones T3 and T4. Effects include autoimmune thyroiditis (Divi at al., 1997, 1996) and hypothyroidism involving obesity, dry skin and hair, low blood pressure, slow pulse, depressed muscular activity, intolerance to cold, goiter, and sluggishness of all physiological functions.

Eating estrogenic foods may increase that risk for estrogen-dependent cancers.

"A woman's own estrogens are a very significant risk factor for breast cancer" (Doerge, Sheehan .et al,; National Center For Toxicological Research 1998).

In 1996, researchers found that women consuming soy protein isolate had increased epithelial hyperplasia, a precursor of malignancies (Petrakis et al).

In 1997, a research study showed that consumption of genistein, a soy isoflavone, caused breast cells to enter into the malignant cell cycle (Dees et al).

Soy is known to alter the menstrual cycle length (Cassidy et al, 1994).

Continued still . . . believe it or not

Estrogens are known to be able to pass through the placenta. "Development is the most sensitive stage to estrogen toxicity because of the indisputable evidence of a wide variety of frank malformations and serious functional deficits in experimental animals and humans" (Sheehan, Doerge, 1998).

Genestein causes alterations in leutinizing hormone regulation, which may cause abnormal brain and reproductive tract development (Faber and Hughes, 1993).

When exposed to estrogen, 50% of human female offspring displayed one or more malformations in the reproductive tract (Sheehan, Doerge, 1998).

Babies on soy infant formula have estradiol levels 13,000–22,000 times higher than babies on milk-based infant formula. "Infants exclusively fed soy infant formula receive the estrogenic equivalent of at least five birth control pills a day" (Irvine et al, 1998).

In male infants, the estrogenic effects of soy interrupt the testosterone surge that occurs in the first few months when testosterone levels can be as high as an adult male. Interruption may cause inhibition of male characteristics and sexual organs (Ross, R.K. et al).

In female infants, the estrogenic effects of soy may speed the rate of maturation. Girls enter puberty earlier than normal: 1% show signs of maturation, including pubic hair and breast development, before the age of three; 14.7% of Caucasian and 50% African American by age eight. Dietary estrogens have been linked as a possible cause of this early development (Herman-Giddens, Marcia E. et al.).

Soy consumption causes decreased testosterone levels in men. Buddhist monks ate tofu to reduce libido. (Of course, there's always Viagra . . .)

Soy consumption has been clearly linked to higher risk of vascular dementia, or Alzheimer's, in men (White et al, 1996). The isoflavones of soy inhibit the enzyme conversion of testosterone to estradiol via the aromatase enzyme necessary for male brain function and maintenance (Irvine, 1998).

Soy is not a complete protein. Like all legumes, it lacks the sulfur containing amino acids cysteine and methionine. Lysine, essential for brain development and maintenance, is denatured during processing.

Still more bad news . . .

Soybeans contain haemagglutinins, a clot-promoting substance that causes red blood cells to clump together.

Soy protein isolate (SPI), the main ingredient in most imitation meat and dairy products, goes through rigorous processing to remove inherent "anti-nutrients." Soybeans are first mixed with an alkaline solution to eliminate fiber then separated using an acid wash and finally neutralized in an alkaline solution. The precipitated curd is spray dried at high temperatures to produce a high protein powder. To make texturized vegetable protein (TVP), this product is further extruded under high temperature and high pressure, creating carcinogenic nitrates from the denaturation of the original protein structure. Often, flavorings containing MSG, a powerful neurotoxin, are added under the guise of "natural flavors."

The only comparatively "safe" soy includes its fermented forms of miso, natto and tempeh. Fermentation—and fermentation only—largely neutralizes trypsin inhibitors and phytic acid. Goitrogens or thyroid inhibitors, however, remain intact even following fermentation, so care must be taken to not over-consume even these soy foods.

See more extensive bibliography and visit the exhaustively-referenced and informative Web site: www.soyonlineservice.co.nz, in addition to www.Mercola.com and www.WestonAPrice.org.

DIGESTION AND NUTRIENT ASSIMILATION:
A NORTH-TO-SOUTH JOURNEY

A person can literally consume the most expensive, best quality source foods there are and still experience illness or marginal health and symptoms. How can this be? One possible and critically important key is digestion. If you can't break down and appropriately assimilate what you eat, at best you are wasting your money on grocery bills. At worst, you are generating rancid, fermented, putrefied and toxic compounds that can reap havoc on every organ and system in your body. Quality digestion cannot be under-rated—and is a subject commonly overlooked when discussing a healthy diet. Every part of the body and mind depends to the extreme on proper digestion to supply it with nutrients necessary for functioning.

Poor digestion is an epidemic problem, as soaring sales of acid-blocking or neutralizing medications, gall-bladder removals and appendectomies neatly illustrate. According to Jonathon Wright, MD, after using Heidelberg Gastro telemetry equipment to examine the stomach pH of thousands of his patients, approximately 90% of Americans produce too little hydrochloric acid (HCl). The implications of this are staggering.

A lack of adequate HCl means several rather major things:

1) Poor digestion and absorption of proteins or amino acids necessary for more than 50,000 functions in the body, including neurotransmitter production for regulation of mood, maintenance and

repair of cells, organs, bone and tissues and many other indispensable functions.

2) Poor absorption of key minerals, including calcium, magnesium, phosphorous, boron, iron and zinc (the double jeopardy here is that it actually also *takes* zinc to make HCl—leading to potentially severe deficiencies of these incredibly important minerals and all that it implies).

3) Poor HCl production by parietal cells in the stomach also impairs proper B12 digestion essential for neurological health. This impairment also can lead to under-secretion of intrinsic factor essential to B12's absorption in the gut. B12 is a key methyl donor necessary for cardiovascular and brain health. We also use it to make red blood cells. Prolonged deficiencies of B12 can result in irreversible neurological damage, severe mood dysregulation, cognitive functioning and dementia, as well as macrocytic anemia and heart disease. Not pretty.

4) The poorly digested mass of rotting chyme in the stomach (sorry to be so graphic) goes on to reap havoc elsewhere in the digestive tract, fermenting and being partially expelled as reflux symptoms, gas and bloating. It generates irritation and inflammation in the small intestine. This can eventually lead to mucosal and microvilli erosion and what can be termed "leaky gut syndrome," a hyper-porosity of the otherwise selectively-permeable membrane of the small intestine where poorly digested proteins may then enter the bloodstream and be treated as antigens or foreign invaders by the immune system, initially resulting in allergies and/or food sensitivities, and possibly even becoming autoimmune disorders.

5) Enhanced vulnerability to parasites and other food-borne illness.

Going from bad to worse . . .

There is one more unpleasant possibility here: if hydrochloric acid deficiency is allowed to become chronic, overgrowth of a normally benign denizen of our GI tract, H. pylori, can occur. In an under-acidic environment in the stomach, H. pylori can begin undesirably proliferating, leading to infiltration of the gut lining, suppression of parietal cells—making HCl production even more difficult—and inflammation or even ulceration of endothelial tissue. This can potentially generate gastritis and ulcers. Additionally, H. pylori may even spread to other endothelial tissue; infiltrating and inflaming arterial endothelium as a now known vector for vascular disease.

We do need *some H. pylori*, however. It plays a complex role in the regulation of leptin, so fully eradicating it is not the answer. Managing excess overgrowth, with certain nutrients and restoring normal hydrochloric acid levels, is the better alternative.

The more difficult to digest a particular protein is, the more excessive the amount of food in a meal, the more overcooked and denatured the protein in that meal is . . . then the more ineffectual or strained hydrochloric acid production will be, and the more likely it will be to cause problems. Gluten in wheat, rye, spelt and oats; casein in especially pasteurized milk and milk products; albumen in chicken eggs; heavily processed soy protein, and overly cooked, denatured proteins in general are all potentially problematic for many and make HCl's job much harder. Overeating is also a total set-up for inadequate digestion. Addressing these issues alone can often correct digestive problems and what may otherwise seem to be HCl insufficiency.

So . . . why don't I have enough HCl?

There are many reasons for hydrochloric acid insufficiency. HCl is produced only in the presence of proteins and is inhibited by sugars and starches. High carbohydrate diets—particularly when combined with inadequate intake of dietary protein, such as in vegetarian/vegan diets—are an extremely common cause of hydrochloric acid insufficiency. Thyroid hypofunction (a low-functioning thyroid) suppresses *gastrin* production—a hormone necessary for signaling HCl production. Certain nutrient deficiencies can also be culprits (B1, zinc and C are needed for HCl production), as well as overeating at meals, inappropriate food combination, excess alcohol consumption, and chronic stress, and anxiety and over-arousal, particularly at mealtime.

Proper hydrochloric acid production is key to the rest of the digestive process, so it's an extremely important issue to address and among the most common deficiencies impacting health.

How it's all *supposed* to work: digestion 101

Bear with me here . . . understanding how digestion naturally works is hugely important!

Remember that *digestion begins in the brain* and that it is a *parasympathetic* process, meaning the body and mind must be in a relaxed, calm state for digestion to properly occur. Eating while rushed, otherwise preoccupied, or stressed, paralyzes normal digestive function and inhibits necessary secretions. It's a great set-up for reflux and indigestion.

Always wait to eat until you have time to relax and focus on the meal . . . take in the aroma of the food, and *take the time to chew.* Amylase in the mouth begins the digestion of carbohydrates, and the food needs to mix in the mouth thoroughly. Poorly chewed food creates far more work for the stomach and requires more HCl to do the same job of breaking down the protein. Chew, chew, *chew!* (Sorry to say, you're mother was right . . . about *that,* anyway.)

From there, the chewed food, or chyme, travels down the esophagus, enters the stomach where it secretes self-protective mucous, and mixes with pepsin and HCl to break down complex proteins into shorter chains, or peptides. Peptides are then further refined by pancreatic enzymes into di- and tri-peptide complexes and amino acids for absorption in the small intestine.

An extremely acid pH—roughly 0.8, almost pure acid—signals

to the pyloric valve (the gateway to the stomach) that preliminary healthy digestion is complete and, like a key, the proper pH opens the valve and allows the happily digested contents to empty into the duodenum. Improper pH signaling (i.e., inadequate hydrochloric acid) can delay this gastric emptying, sometimes for hours, resulting in the fermentation of stomach contents and potentially generating reflux symptoms.

Try this experiment at home: take a blender and throw some meat in it, some potatoes, some Pepsi (you might substitute a glass of wine), some ketchup, sour cream (for the potatoes), bread rolls and butter and . . . what the heck, why not dessert? Now blend it all together, spit in it, then put it in a room that is 98.6 degrees for an hour or two (or more). I'll leave the results to your imagination.

Improperly digested chyme becomes rancid, putrefied and ferments to become toxic compounds that the body, via the gatekeeper—the pyloric valve, is reluctant to allow through. When the pyloric valve (between the stomach and small intestine) is locked tight and won't let the food continue down, sometimes the contents will simply back up. *Voila*—reflux!

The stomach is an acid organ. It thrives in the presence of extreme acid when healthy, and its contents *must be acidic enough!*

Even less-than-adequately-acidic gastric pH can feel extremely acidic to the delicate esophagus, which has zero protection from acid, during reflux . . . but just think of what you're doing when you use an acid blocker or neutralizer to treat this symptom. Acid reflux is nearly always a consequence of not enough stomach acid, rather than too much! Short-term relief of symptoms by chronically using something that neutralizes stomach acid can lead to long term disaster! These drugs were *never* meant to be used long term. Adequate hydrochloric acid is essential for the proper digestion of proteins, at least fourteen different minerals, vitamin B12 and, to some degree, folic acid.

It's also essential to the proper execution of the rest of the entire digestive process.

Having inadequate HCl can be a real problem.

Gas, bloating, belching and a feeling of heaviness in the stomach after meals are all classic symptoms of inadequate hydrochloric acid production, as is reflux. Weak, brittle nails or, in some, excessive hair loss can also be common symptoms. They represent only the tip of the much bigger iceberg.

Meanwhile . . . Further South:

At the same time the appropriately acidic chyme enters the duodenum, the proper pH signals the production of protective mucous to protect the vulnerable duodenum from stomach acids. The hormone *secretin* then signals the pancreas to release both bicarbonate (to neutralize the stomach acid so the next phase of digestion can occur) and pancreatic enzymes to further digest the food particles.

Another hormone that senses the presence of fats, *cholecystekinin,* or CCK, stimulates the gallbladder to release bile into the bile duct, which then empties into the duodenum where it can emulsify the fats there into smaller globules for easier assimilation. Bile function is also influenced by gastric pH signaling. Poor bile function can thwart this part of the process, leading to incomplete digestion of fats, poor fat-soluble nutrient assimilation, and ultimately deficiencies of these vital key nutrients. Trust me when I say this is a bad, *bad* thing.

Bile can become stagnant and unhealthy for many reasons, though the most common culprits include poor hydrochloric acid production, over-consumption of processed fats, rancid fats, trans fats, excess estrogens or an excessively low-fat diet. You see, bile is normally very watery in its consistency and is composed of mainly cholesterol (yes . . . *eeevil* cholesterol), bile salts, phospholipids, certain minerals, other nutrients, bile pigments and taurine. Bad (i.e., processed, rancid or artificial) fats or stagnating bile from disuse, as via low-fat diets, can alter its consistency, thickening it and making it's expulsion from the gallbladder sluggish, painful or nearly impossible. Stagnant bile may then begin to precipitate out cholesterol, pigments or calcium as small, or not-so-small stones.

Heaven forbid one of these stones should attempt to traverse through or occlude the bile duct and then you eat a bucket of the Colonel's "Secret Recipe." This can trigger a nasty gallbladder attack and send you unceremoniously to the hospital, where doctors will be only too eager to surgically part you from your gallbladder forever. Sometimes doctors recommend removing gallbladders preemptively or even (as insane as this is), "preventatively," even where there is nothing wrong with it . . . *"yet."*

Don't be fooled into thinking you don't really need your gallbladder, though they may try to convince you that you don't. Living without a gallbladder can lead to lifelong issues with inadequate fat and fat-soluble nutrient digestion, deficiencies, fatigue, hormonal imbalances and other problems. Carefully and systematically restoring biliary health should be a first choice wherever reasonably possible.

Taking bile salts with every fat-containing meal is a must in the absence of having a functional gallbladder. Additionally, care must be taken that one does not develop deficiencies of essential fatty acids (EFAs) and vitamins A, D, E and K.

Poor pH in the stomach and/or biliary problems further north along the digestive journey set the stage for irritable bowel syndrome (IBS), duodenal ulcers, yeast overgrowth, vulnerability to parasites and other food-borne illness, dysbiosis, imbalances of healthy gastrointestinal flora or "healthy bacteria," the "Big C" (constipation) and even ultimately worse problems.

Suffice it to say, it is not a happy ending. (No pun intended.)

Yikes! What do I do?

So much can be accomplished toward optimizing proper digestion by following a few simple guidelines:

▶ Take time out and focus on being relaxed and calmly present at mealtime

▶ Chew, chew, chew!

▶ Minimize fluid intake at meals. Stick to only small sips of water and avoid other beverages

▶ Consume high quality protein, not soy, cooked as minimally as possible (except, of course, chicken and pork) in small to moderate quantities at mealtime

▶ Avoid combining proteins with starches and sugars, even fruit, at mealtime. Stick to fibrous, non-starchy vegetables and greens

▶ Consider the incorporation of quality lacto-fermented foods and raw, cultured vegetables with meals. These can help restore healthy bacteria and provide many enzymes that may assist in the digestive process. They are especially helpful when one is eating a lot of otherwise cooked and denatured foods. They are also delicious.

▶ Do not fear naturally occurring fat or get suckered into eating a low-fat diet. Remember, we are designed to eat fat, and a significant amount of it. This is why we have a gallbladder in the first place. We're creatures of the Ice Age—remember? Use it or lose it.

Important note: The only exception here is a person who may be experiencing gallbladder symptoms (gallbladder attacks, aching pain under the right side of the rib cage, especially to the touch, and/or nausea at meals), in which case this should be dealt with cautiously, and a low-fat diet may be entirely appropriate until the issue is resolved. Consult with a qualified healthcare provider. Remember, don't be a hero . . . and don't push it. *Listen to your body.*

▶ Avoid non-fermented soy (a topic covered more exhaustively elsewhere in this book). Soy contains enzyme inhibitors, which can ruin your ability to digest and absorb protein over time.

For some, taking hydrochloric acid as a supplement at mealtime may be appropriate and necessary for a time, until your stomach is able to resume its own production. If you experience gas, bloating or excessive fullness after meals, the rule is: start with one capsule of HCl with your meal. If you do not experience a "slight warming sensation" with that, take two with your next meal . . . and so on until a sensation of warming is achieved. Then back off by one capsule, and that is your dose. The amount of protein in the meal should be used as a gauge with dosing. (In other words, don't take a handful of HCl capsules if all you're having is one or two lonely shrimp on your salad.) This process tends to be self-weaning, and your stomach will usually tell you when you need to start backing off.

Eventually, your stomach should be able to restore appropriate HCl production on its own. If it doesn't, there may be some other underlying problem, such as *H. pylori* overgrowth, poorly functioning thyroid or some other issue. Seek out a Nutritional Therapy Practitioner (NTP), Certified Nutritional Therapist (CNT) or some other natural healthcare provider for evaluation.

The exceptions to undertaking HCl supplementation are those people with ulcers, gastritis or a current, acute reflux problem. The inflamed gastric and esophageal tissue needs to heal before sufferers should start taking HCl supplements. This can be accomplished with supplements containing deglycyrrhizinated (DGL) licorice, vitamin U (or lots of very fresh, raw cabbage juice), vitamins A and D, high strength mucopolysaccharide-rich organic aloe vera and L-glutamine.

Pancreatic enzymes, taken on an empty stomach, can further assist in digestion for those who lack adequate natural production. Consumption of smaller, more easily digested meals, avoiding soy foods, as well as other legumes and grains, and increasing normalization of HCl and gastric pH, can also contribute to normalization of pancreatic output.

Some individuals have a deficiency of an important pancreatic fat-digesting enzyme called *lipase*. Lipase deficiency may be more prevalent in those prone to diabetes and glucose dysregulation. Taking lipase, as part of a pancreatic enzyme supplement, on an empty stomach throughout the day can help restore healthy fat digestion for some and make eliminating the dependence upon sugar as your primary source of fuel much easier.

Those experiencing biliary stasis or who may have cholesterol-type gallstones may benefit from taking a couple of tablespoons of raw apple cider vinegar with their meals. The malic acid can help soften the stones and thin the bile over time. Other biliary support may include beet juice (of mainly tops and stems), taurine, and phosphatidyl choline supplementation for helping thin bile and restore better biliary function. Phosphoric acid supplements can be helpful with dissolving calcium-type gallstones.

Remember—everything begins and ends with proper digestion. Improving this alone can be a miracle to many!

YOUR GUT AND THE IMMUNE CONNECTION

Few people are aware that between 70% and 80% of our immune system resides in our gut. The mucosal layer, a mere single cell in thickness, serves as the superficial veil for the gut-associated lymphatic tissue (GALT). It is the first line of defense in our immune system and clusters of cells there, known as Peyer's patches, along with secretory IgA (SIgA), located in the mucosa and also located protectively on the surface of lung tissue, are the sentinels that alert both T- and B-cells to possible invasion of unwanted antigens and microbes. Stress, excessively low or high cortisol, infection and poor diet can strip secretory IgA from the gut and lungs, rendering it extremely vulnerable. The primary food for enterocytes (the cells of the small intestine)is the amino acid L-glutamine. Added supplementation, along with maintaining healthy dietary guidelines outlined here, can enhance and help facilitate more rapid regeneration of eroded gastrointestinal mucosa and depleted secretory IgA levels, though this can still take time.

"There are more bacteria in our intestinal tract than cells in our body."
—Jeffery Bland, Ph.D

Gastrointestinal flora, or healthy bacteria, are also an undeniably important part of this equation. Few individuals today maintain healthy populations of these vital GI denizens, which outnumber all other cells in the human body combined! There are literally hundreds of probiotic species, most of which are, as yet, little researched or understood. The most common varieties include lactobacillus (found primarily in the small intestine), bifidobacteria (found primarily in the large intestine), bacteroides, eubacterium, peptococcaceae, streptococcus, ruminococcus and fusobacteria. They may be either aerobic or anaerobic in nature.

These probiotic species are commonly established at birth via the birth canal and breast milk, and they colonize very quickly in infancy. In babies whose GI probiotic colonization is poor there is a greater tendency toward colic, gas, and diaper rash, as well as development of allergy, asthma, and eczema. Early problems with GI integrity and healthy colonization are also exceedingly common in autism.

Our ancestors also obtained soil-based organisms through natural exposure to dirt on food. This has recently been hypothesized to have been an important dietary source of beneficial flora lacking in today's more antiseptic food preparation methods. (Note, however, that I do not advocate eating unwashed produce today because of this.)

Most of us carry three to four pounds of bacteria in our gut at any given time. Ideally, at least 85% should be of the friendly variety; no more than 15% should be of the less favorable kind. These bacteria help convert fiber and other indigestible material to usable nutrients, facilitate the absorption of certain minerals, assist in detoxification, and maintain and protect the gastrointestinal mucosa. They may also help in the prevention of allergies, skin disorders, inflammatory bowel disease, ear infections, vaginitis, bladder infections, constipation and diarrhea. Probiotics have more recently been demonstrated in studies to modulate immune responses via the gut's mucosal immune system. Certain exogenously derived soil-based organisms (SBOs) have also been hypothesized to be a more natural part of our ancient diets and may be uniquely beneficial in restoring gut health for some. They may be purchased in supplement form, as well.

Most probiotic supplements commercially sold tend to be of questionable viability, though there are exceptions. The brands available via healthcare practitioners may be somewhat more reliable, in this regard, where production tends to more rigorously adhere to certain standards. Probiotic supplementation is probably a good idea for most people. These are best taken on an empty stomach at least a half hour prior to meals, though instructions may vary from brand to brand. Steer clear of budget brands. I recommend cycling through different quality brands, giving your gut a variety of strains and potencies. These tend to work synergistically.

The most effective and inexpensive solution to restore healthy gastrointestinal flora, by far, includes the addition of raw, lacto-fermented vegetables and, if tolerated, homemade raw, milk-based kefir and yogurt to the diet. This suggestion does *not* include conventional, commercial forms of kefir and yogurt sold in grocery stores, however. Pasteurized milk is a source of countless problems for many, if not most people. Conventional, store-bought kefir and yogurt tend to contain extremely high levels of carbohydrates and undesirable additives. Learning to make your own from quality raw cow, sheep or goat's milk is easy. (See *Nourishing Traditions* by Sally Fallon.)

Perhaps the single most acutely damaging impact on the balance of gastrointestinal flora involves the use—particularly the extended use—of antibiotics. (There goes the intestinal neighborhood!) Reverberations can continue for many, many years beyond a single course of antibiotics, and re-establishing healthy GI flora can be extremely difficult, particularly after the "bad guys" have moved in and taken hold. For this reason alone, antibiotics should only be used when absolutely and undeniably essential—which is rarely the case. If you absolutely cannot avoid the use of antibiotics, take care to supplement your diet with quality and abundant probiotics both during and after using antibiotics for up to several weeks or months, to help prevent long term complications and common secondary infections.

The second brain?

Although serotonin is a neurotransmitter widely associated with the brain and mood functioning—including the prevention of depression, anxiety and insomnia—few are aware that 95% of all serotonin production in the body lies not in the brain but in the gut.

The gut, in fact, has even more neurons than the brain! The next time you find yourself struggling with mood issues, consider first the quality of your GI health and digestion. The brain and gut are inextricably linked.

DIETARY FATS:
THE GOOD, THE BAD AND THE UGLY

The commonly held belief that the best diet for prevention of coronary heart disease is a low saturated fat, low cholesterol diet is not supported by the available evidence from clinical trials.
—*EUROPEAN HEART JOURNAL*, Volume 18, January 1997

Even though the focus of dietary recommendations is usually a reduction of saturated fat intake, no relation between saturated fat intake and risk of coronary heart disease was observed in the most informative prospective study to date.
—WILLETT, 1990, Harvard University

Dietary fat has a little-deserved and much-maligned recent history in the popular press. Yet a diet moderately high in both saturated and monounsaturated fats and certain essential polyunsaturated fats such as omega-3s has been ongoing in our history spanning nearly a hundred thousand generations.

What changed?

The multifold answer lies in the abundance of refined carbohydrates in the modern diet: highly poly-unsaturated vegetable oils (these are new to the human diet and containing predominantly omega-6 fatty acids, which are essential but excessively present in modern diets and may cause serious imbalances), grain or corn-fed meats, farmed sea foods, also rich in excess omega-6 fatty acids and having very little omega-3s, and hydrogenated and partially hydrogenated oils.

Cooking with such oils promotes carcinogenicity, inflammation and unhealthy imbalances of fatty acids in the body. The excess omega-6, omega-9 and trans fats also exacerbate insulin resistance. Trans fats—that is, hydrogenated or partially-hydrogenated fats and oils found in margarine spreads, vegetable shortening, commercial vegetable oils (particularly soybean and canola), salad dressings, baked or packaged goods, and virtually all fast foods—are created in a laboratory, not in nature. They most certainly do not belong in our diets.

Care must also be taken to make sure the animal fat consumed comes from clean, grass-fed-only organic sources (i.e., pesticide-free, hormone-free, etc.). Many toxins are, in fact, fat-soluble and readily stored in animal body-fat. Meat consumed from grain or corn-fed animals should probably be as lean and trimmed of fat as possible or countered with extra omega-3 supplementation, and always organic. High, imbalanced levels of omega-6 in grain and corn-fed meats tend to promote inflammatory processes, insulin resistance and interference with omega-3 metabolism. *Exclusively* grass-fed meat is vastly preferable though harder to come by, and the fat in such meat is rich in desirable omega-3 and conjugated linoleic acid (CLA)—both highly beneficial fats.

We are creatures of the Ice Age.

This is hugely important to remember. Fat, to all humans, means "survival" to our physiological functioning. Diets low in fat paradoxically cause the body to more easily synthesize fat from other sources, most notably, carbohydrates, and absorb and store this unwanted fat. Diets high in carbohydrates trigger our master hormone, leptin, to become severely dysregulated. Blood sugar surges lead to leptin surges—and ultimately to leptin resistance, in which leptin signaling is no longer effectively heard by the brain. This sends a message of "starva-tion" to the hypothalamus, which then reacts promptly with increases in appetite or cravings and inspires unhealthy binge eating.

Low-fat diets, often replete with empty carbohydrates, have re-sulted in little more than accelerated weight gain in many, significant essential nutrient deficiencies, uninspiring menu selections, general frustration and feelings of deprivation. Nothing has contributed to our obesity epidemic more.

Moderate natural dietary fat is only potentially problematic or "fattening" in the presence of dietary carbohydrate.

Our more primitive ancestors sought out and ate plenty of qual-ity fat, including saturated fat and cholesterol, containing ample amounts of critical fat soluble nutrients—*up to ten times our modern day intake.* They suffered none of our modern afflictions, including heart disease, diabetes, cancer or obesity. It's no paradox.

In Framingham, Massachusetts, the more saturated fat one ate, the more cholesterol one ate, the more calories one ate, the lower people's serum cholesterol. We found that the people who ate the most cholesterol, ate the most saturated fat, ate the most calories weighed the least and were the most physically active.
—From *Archives of Internal Medicine,* 1992, DR. WILLIAM CASTILLI, Director of the Framingham Study

Reduced fat and caloric intake and frequent use of low caloric food prod-ucts have been associated with a paradoxical increase in the prevalence of obesity.
—HEINI AF; WEINSIER RL. "Divergent trends in obesity and fat intake patterns: the American paradox." American Journal of Medi-cineet al.et al 1997 Mar., 102(3): *259–64*

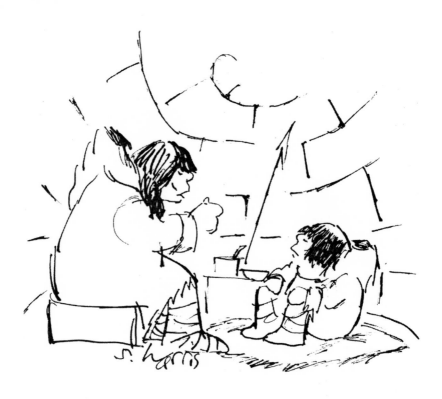

"EVERY DAY YOU SHOULD EAT SOMETHING FROM EACH OF THE FIVE BASIC FOOD GROUPS: FRIED BLUBBER, BOILED BLUBBER, STEWED BLUBBER, BAKED BLUBBER AND RAW BLUBBER."

The idea that saturated fats cause heart disease is completely wrong, but the statement has been "published" so many times over the last three or more decades that it is very difficult to convince people otherwise unless they are willing to take the time to read and learn what produced the "anti-saturated fat agenda.

—DR. MARY ENIG, consulting editor to *The Journal of the American College of Nutrition,* President of the Maryland Nutritionists Association and world-renowned lipids researcher

Consider the following:

► The French eat more saturated fats in the form of meat, liver, pâté, butter, cream, and cheese than people in almost any other Western nation, yet heart-related death rate among middle-aged men in France is 145 per 100,000, compared to 315 per 100,000 in America. Heart-related deaths in France are actually *lowest* in Gascony, the region of France where people eat the most fat

► Most people think the Japanese eat a low-fat diet, but this is a myth. The truth is that they get plenty of fat from eggs, chicken, beef, pork, organ meats and shellfish. The amount of animal fat in their diet has gone up steadily since World War II—yet rates of heart disease there are among the lowest in the world and their average lifespan has actually increased

► Scientists in India discovered that people in the northern part of the country ate seventeen times more animal fat than people in the south, but their overall incidence of heart disease was **seven times lower**

The bottom line here is that your body needs saturated fat and cholesterol and is designed to make use of it.

> **Saturated fat and cholesterol are not the culprits in heart disease!**

Keep in mind, also, that all fats differ substantially from one another in their biochemical structure, in the way they are digested and absorbed, and in their specific physiological effects. They also may behave differently, even among individual types, depending on what other foods are consumed with them.

There are several different forms of saturated fat, in fact; short, medium and long-chained varieties are utilized in the body in very different ways. Some are readily used for energy; others are more apt to be stored. You can never just use the term "fat" and encompass this myriad of differences in their biological activity.

Perhaps the biggest misconception of all is that all fat is basically the same—or even that all saturated fat is the same. Natural dietary fats function with intricate complexity in the human body, and they are needed and utilized in varied ways under varied circumstances.

The fact is that all natural fats have a role to play in our health and what matters in the end is proper balance. Artificial, overly processed or rancid fats, however, are the ones that need to be avoided altogether.

DISPELLING THE CHOLESTEROL MYTH

Besides real diseases we are subject to many that are only imaginary, for which the physicians have invented imaginary cures; these have then several names, and so have the drugs that are proper for them.
—Jonathan Swift (1667–1745)

Cholesterol is a vital substance in the human body. Using cholesterol, the body produces a series of stress-combating hormones and mediates the health and efficiency of the cell membranes. Cholesterol is found in the nerve sheaths, the white matter of the brain and the adrenal glands. It also helps regulate the body's electrolyte balance. It is regarded by the body as such an important metabolic aid that every cell has a mechanism to manufacture its own supply (Erdmann, 1995).

Cholesterol is also essential for brain function and development. It forms membranes inside cells and keeps cell membranes permeable. It keeps moods level by stabilizing neurotransmitters and helps maintain a healthy immune system. No steroidal hormone can be manufactured without it, including estrogen, progesterone, testosterone, adrenaline, cortisol and dehydroepiandrosterone (DHEA).

Up to two grams, or 2000 mg, of cholesterol are produced internally every day, several times the amount found in our diets. *Despite this ability to manufacture cholesterol, it is, in fact, critical to obtain cholesterol from dietary sources.* The human diet has always contained significant amounts of it. Restricting or eliminating its intake indicates a crisis or famine to the body . The result is the production of a liver enzyme called *HMG-CoA reductase* that, in effect, then overproduces cholesterol from carbohydrates in the diet. Consuming excess carbohydrates while decreasing cholesterol intake guarantees a steady overproduction of cholesterol in the body. The only way to switch this overproduction off is to consume an adequate amount of dietary cholesterol and back off the carbs. In other words, the *dietary intake of cholesterol stops the internal production of cholesterol* (Schwarzbein, 1999).

Most "statin" drugs used to lower cholesterol are designed to inhibit the action of HMG-CoA reductase artificially at the dangerous and costly expense of depleting the body's own Coenzyme Q10 reserves. *CoQ10 may be the single most important nutrient for the functioning of the heart.* Furthermore, statins have never even been proven to lessen the risk of a heart attack.

A sobering aside: political commentator Tim Russert was taking statin drugs at the time of his death. Tragically, he was prescribed these drugs even though his cholesterol was completely normal. His doctors had put him on statins "preventatively." There is talk today of similarly prescribing statins "preventatively" to children. A new report shows the number of kids taking statin drugs has sharply risen 68% in just five years. We simply cannot, in our right minds, allow this to happen!

Study after study has demonstrated the potentially debilitating effects of statin drugs. They can produce confused states similar to Alzheimer's disease. A new study published in the *Journal of the American College of Cardiology* revealed that driving down cholesterol levels actually *increases* the risk of cancer (Alawi et al, 2007).

Among the many potential side effects of statin use includes:

- Depression
- Confusion
- Inability to concentrate
- Amnesia
- Disorientation
- Weakened immune system
- Increased risk of cancer
- Shortness of breath
- Liver damage
- Fatigue
- CoQ10 depletion/deficiency and weakening of the heart
- Lowered sex drive
- Impotence
- Kidney failure
- Nerve pain
- Muscle weakness
- Rhabdomyolysis (painful deterioration/destruction of muscle cells)
- Death

By conveniently placing the blame on low-density lipoprotein (LDL) cholesterol, nothing is done to address the actual underlying problems that cause heart disease. Fully 50-75% of those who have heart attacks have what doctors term "normal cholesterol." (My own father, a prominent medical doctor and the man who literally wrote a textbook entitled *Radiological Cardiology,* was one of them.)

The best approach for anyone wanting to prevent heart disease is a normal, unrestricted dietary intake of cholesterol and healthy natural fat, total avoidance of highly processed or rancid vegetable oils and trans fats, and *a reduced or eliminated starch and sugar-based carbohydrate intake.*

Dietary cholesterol may, in fact, be additionally beneficial to the gastrointestinal lining, where it improves cell-membrane integrity and can help prevent excessive permeability.

The bottom line is that we are fully designed, and well suited, for consuming and healthfully metabolizing naturally occurring cholesterol. Cholesterol is not our enemy.

No study to date has adequately shown any significant link between dietary and serum cholesterol levels . . . *or any significant causative link between cholesterol and actual heart disease.* Other than in uncommon cases of genetically based familial hypercholesterolemia— where natural mechanisms which regulate cholesterol production fail and the body cannot stop overproduction (and even here the proof of the problematic nature of cholesterol is dubious, at best)—cholesterol is perhaps only potentially deleterious in and of itself in oxidized forms, occurring as a result of food processing methods, such as in reduced-fat milks, powdered milk or eggs, and high-heat cooking or frying.

Inflammatory processes can also be oxidizing of cholesterol in the body. Other than this, *all* cholesterol in the body is the same. High-density lipoproteins (HDL) and low-density lipoproteins (LDL) only reflect transport mechanisms for healthy cholesterol and are meaningless measures of coronary heart disease risk (Enig, Ravnskov, 1998).

It is also important to realize that HDL and LDL are not actual cholesterol at all, but merely the protein transport mechanism for cholesterol.

All cholesterol is exactly the same.

LDL takes cholesterol away from the liver to the extremities and other organs for various purposes, and HDL merely returns the same cholesterol to the liver where it may be recycled.

There is one undesirable variation of a certain LDL-carrier molecule known as lipoprotein(a), which is smaller and denser than regular LDL. Within the arterial endothelium lie spaces between cells that serve as channels for the influx and outflow of nutrients. Lipoprotein(a) can actually lodge itself in the spaces between these vascular arterial cells and shut off that natural channel, resulting in poor nutrient flow to the endothelium, stagnation and damaging inflammatory response. Lipoprotein(a) is the only lipoprotein of significant consequence. The drug companies, however, would rather you didn't know about it at all, as statin drugs do nothing to change the size of LDL particles or reduce lipoprotein(a)—*only diet can do this*. It is high carbohydrate diets and the presence of excess insulin that are responsible for the production of this undesirable lipoprotein. Diets rich in natural fats and moderate protein with low carbohydrates have normal LDL. Regular LDL and HDL are of little actual consequence, though they can serve as a relative marker for illuminating certain dietary tendencies. They may also in part reflect other disorders and may be useful to look at in that regard.

Furthermore, cholesterol is the human body's version of duct tape. It travels to areas where there has been arterial damage and patches up lesions. Higher serum levels of cholesterol may serve as a message that "something is going on" for which it is needed. It is simply an indicator, *not* a "diagnosis."

Going in with statin drugs to stamp out cholesterol is the equivalent of preventing the firemen who arrive to put out a fire from doing their job—and blaming them for the fire. Elevated glucose and/or insulin levels, for instance, damage arterial walls and lead to an increased need for cholesterol to repair them.

Roughly 80%, of what actually clogs arteries is not even composed of cholesterol or saturated fat but of oxidized or rancid *unsaturated* fats (Enig). Statistically, individuals whose blood cholesterol levels are low develop just as many plaques in their blood vessels as individuals whose cholesterol is "high" (Ravnskov, 1998).

Cholesterol is no more a cause of heart disease than gray hair is the cause of old age.

Cholesterol

☺

Framingham data—thirty-year observation

	Cholesterol mg/dl 205-234	235-265
Men		Deaths/1000
Age 35-44	3	6
45-54	11	11
55-64	20	21
65-74	22	23
35-64 (age adjusted)	13	14
Women		
Age 35-44	1	1
45-54	4	2
55-64	8	7
65-74	11	13
35-64 (age adjusted)	5	4

Many are unaware that cholesterol is also an antioxidant or that levels too low (below 150mg/dL) are linked with aggressive or suicidal behavior, and cause mortality and increase cancer risk. I, personally, worry far more about someone with cholesterol levels that are too low than too high. In addition, normal hormonal production and balance is utterly dependent on the availability of cholesterol in the body. Cholesterol is the primary building block of many hormones. It is also essential for normal cognitive functioning and brain development. *We cannot live or function optimally without it.*

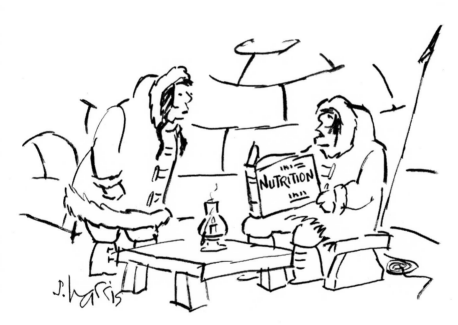

"IT APPEARS THAT OUR DIET IS ALMOST ONE HUNDRED PERCENT CHOLESTEROL. THAT APPEARS TO BE VERY, VERY, VERY BAD."

Comparison of the amount of cholesterol eaten per day by patients with coronary heart disease (CHD) and age- and sex-matched control individuals in ten studies:

Cholesterol eaten per day, in MG

		Patients with CHD	Healthy Subjects
Male Chicago workers		721	757
Framingham citizens	men	708	716
	women	520	477
Puerto Rican men	urban	449	442
	rural	335	358
Puerto Ricans		419	417
Honolulu citizens		549	555
Men from Zutphen, The Netherlands		446	429
Irish men from Ireland and the US		854	832
Citizens from Rancho Bernardo California, USA	men	470	409
	women	226	309
Participants in the LRC study	age 30-59	427	416
	age 60-79	423	355
Hawaiian citizens	Hawaiian men	510	680
	Japanese men	466	587

"Perhaps the biggest obstacle to a more rational debate about cholesterol, heart disease, or any other health problem, is the simple fact that too many of the people we turn to for advice on such matters—our doctors—are tied to the makers of drugs. Sometimes those ties involve several hundred thousand dollars a year, sometimes just a few warm doughnuts."
—Ray Moynihan and Alan Cassels, from *Selling Sickness,* 2005

Furthermore . . . It is an interesting irony that many of the most vital, protective and supportive nutrients promoted for cardiovascular health in their most utilizable forms are those found (either richly, predominantly or exclusively) in animal-source foods or best absorbed from them, and are typically rich in fat, cholesterol and complete proteins. These include Coenzyme Q10, Taurine, EPA and DHA, conjugated linolenic acid (CLA), key glutathione precursor L-cysteine, L-carnitine, vitamins A and D, anti-homocysteine vitamins B6, B12, folic acid (richly abundant in liver), R-Lipoic acid, magnesium, zinc, chromium and sulphur, to name a few.

Saturated fat, particularly 18-carbon stearic acid utilized in the form of ketones, is the preferred fuel for the human heart, liver and kidneys (Enig).

> **Children should never, ever be put on low-fat or low-cholesterol diets.**

Studies have overwhelmingly shown that the younger the child, the more critical fat and cholesterol becomes to the brain and nervous system's development. Breast milk is especially rich in omega-3s, saturated fat and medium-chain triglycerides (MCTs), an important component of some saturated fats, such as coconut oil. Fats are also essential for the absorption of many solely fat-soluble nutrients, such as vitamins A, E, D, and K, as well as the many minerals which rely on such vitamins as co-factors and are necessary for their proper absorption.

The presence of dietary fat is critical for the proper utilization of dietary protein. We need quality natural fat in significant quantities, if not abundance, for the optimal functioning of our bodies and our brains.

The human body and brains' primary source of fuel is designed to be fat in the form of ketones—not glucose!

Critical fat-soluble nutrients, particularly true vitamins A (found only in animal sources) and D, were especially high in primitive and traditional diets—often ten times higher than in modern diets (Price). Beta-carotene, a fat-soluble nutrient, is not, contrary to popular press, the equivalent of vitamin A—nor is its conversion to vitamin A a simple matter. Children under the age of five and individuals with liver or thyroid impairment cannot make this conversion at all.

The conversion also requires the presence of dietary fat. Furthermore, it takes no less than six units of beta-carotene to biochemically form a single unit of vitamin A *(Basic Medical Biochemistry)*. One should never rely solely on vegetable sources for this incredibly vital nutrient. Remember, vitamin A (retinol) is not the same thing as beta-carotene (see below). High vitamin cod liver oil can be an excellent supplemental source of true vitamins A and D (mostly A), as well as some omega-3, and may be additionally helpful in the reversal of mineral deficiencies.

β-Carotene

Vitamin A (retinol)

VITAMIN D . . .
WHAT ALL 'DA BUZZ IS ABOUT

(Vitamin D) may be the single most important organic nutrient for your overall health. In fact, if this were a drug, it would be considered the discovery of the century.
—AL SEARS, M.D. from *Your Best Health Under the Sun*

Vitamin D has gotten quite a bit of press in recent years—and deservedly so. Innumerable studies are touting it as the single greatest preventative nutrient against cancer. Recent studies in Canada, in fact, showed that vitamin D lowered risk of all forms of cancer in women by a remarkable 77%. In men, this figure was closer to 60%.

Vitamin D has also been shown to:

- Greatly reduce inflammation
- Prevents most forms of cancer, including skin cancers
- Prevent autoimmune diseases like multiple sclerosis and rheumatoid arthritis
- Support healthy immune function
- Prevent cardiovascular disease
- Prevent Parkinson's disease
- Help maintain healthy musculoskeletal structure
- Help prevent both type-1 and type-2 diabetes
- Support healthy mood and prevent seasonal affective disorders
- Support brain health

- Be critical for the absorption and utilization of calcium and phosphorus

Plus, this news flash: *Vitamin D is also arguably **the** most potent antioxidant in the body, hands down.*

As much as vitamin E is the primary protective nutrient for omega-6s in nature, vitamin D is similarly the primary antioxidant and protective nutrient for omega-3s in nature (Sullivan, 2006). Vitamin D is also much more an actual steroid hormone than a vitamin.

The unfortunate flaw in nutrient research

All this renewed attention toward such a clearly important and previously undervalued nutrient is, of course, wonderful.

The problem lies in one simple fact: all nutrients operate in a complex system of interrelationships in the body, and requirements will vary greatly from person to person. Furthermore, modern day research simply fails to take all these variables into account, instead studying nutrients in relative isolation, compartmentalizing what is never compartmentalized in nature.

The role of certain nutrients in relation to others and the need for certain co-factors in order to optimize a nutrient's function or prevent imbalances isn't normally discussed at all.

This, of course, leads to problems. For instance—and perhaps critically—for each and every receptor for vitamin D, there are *two* receptors for vitamin A on every cell. Because of the compartmentalized approach to vitamin D research, this sort of thing does not get recognized or discussed. A relative balance of these two nutrients is vital to their healthy function in the body. An excess of one can create a relative deficiency of the other. For instance, if you take large amounts of vitamin D without vitamin A, you are potentially more likely to develop symptoms of vitamin-A deficiency. Conversely, taking certain commercial cod liver oil supplements that are rich in vitamin A but poor in vitamin D can lead to more severe vitamin D deficiencies (Important to read labels. A good amount of vitamin D in a serving of cod liver oil should be around 1,000 IU. One can also add extra D in addition to the cod liver oil if need be). Recent research from Spain indicates that vitamin A is necessary for both vitamin-D binding and vitamin-D release to receptor sites. The two are synergistic and should always be balanced in the diet or in supplementation.

Additionally, vitamin E helps recycle vitamin A, vitamin A needs zinc in order to be properly utilized, zinc and copper need to be in a 8:1 to 12:1 balance in order to function properly . . . and on and on. Inadequate levels of either A or D, coupled with a significantly higher level of one or the other, can also result in a relative toxicity at much lower levels than if the two were properly balanced.

This complex web of interrelationships is rarely discussed in the articles promoting vitamin D, or any other nutrient, as the answer to all ills. This is deeply problematic.

Furthermore, often no mention is made of all the varying requirements for vitamin D relative to individual needs, or time of year. Taking any solitary nutrient doesn't just affect one thing—it affects many, *many* things. This needs to be intelligently considered. Plus, those with impaired biliary function or surgically removed gallbladders may find it particularly difficult to absorb and utilize even supplemental fat soluble nutrients.

Complex systems modeling, functional medicine, and functionally, foundationally-based nutritional therapy must be the next evolution of research and practice across the spectrum of healthcare. Science and medicine can no longer be compartmentalized in their thinking, or sell their souls to pharmaceutical and corporate greed, if we are to genuinely uncover useful truths toward our enhanced well-being.

With all that in mind, back to vitamin D . . .

According to the Vitamin D Council, the amount of vitamin D most of us should have—measured as 25-hydroxyvitamin D, or 25(OH)D, in the blood—in order to prevent cancer is about 60 ng/dL. The recommended range of serum 25(OH)D according to a wide variety of experts lies somewhere between 40 and 80 ng/dL. The optimal amount, in light of the Vitamin D Council's findings, is probably closer to 60 to 80 ng/dL. Currently, it is advised that no one exceed 100–150 ng/dL, as higher levels of D over time can be toxic.

Deficiencies of vitamin A, however, can make vitamin D toxic at much lower levels. Excesses of A can also result in greater vitamin D deficiency. Again, proper balance is needed.

Care must be taken to supplement with a D-complex, containing its numerous co-factors in relative balance, or, rather, with vitamin A in its *true* state: as found in beef liver, butter and what is called "high vitamin" cod liver oil (rich in both A and D)—not simply beta carotene. Don't just take a vitamin D pill. Emulsified, liquid forms of supplemental vitamin D may be a better choice for some, as they are far better absorbed by most and much safer. Emulsification improves water solubility and excesses may be more readily excreted. Since most commercially sold cod liver oil tends to be rich in vitamin A but actually has rather poor vitamin D content, adding some emulsified D to cod liver oil supplementation may be more optimal. For more information on cod liver oil and recommended brands, see: http://westonaprice.org/basicnutrition/cod-liver-oil-menu.html.

It is very difficult to ascertain just how much D to recommend for any given individual, supplementally, to adequately meet their needs. Recommended supplementary amounts of vitamin D may vary from as low as 1,000 IU, for relative maintenance in an otherwise D-sufficient individual, to upwards of 10,000 IU per day or more, for, say, an autoimmune condition or cancer. The American Recommended Daily Allowance, woefully outdated, is a meager 400 IU. Available data from modern day primitive hunter-gatherer societies, estimates that the daily dietary intake was probably close to 4,000 IU of dietary vitamin D per day (Weston Price). This does not include vitamin D synthesized in the body from sun exposure, another highly variable and unpredictable thing. Higher amounts may be needed for a time to remediate deficiency states, however, or for specific conditions.

Your need for D depends on much more than (your geographic location); your skin color, your age, your sunning habits, your diet, your genes, your weather (clouds, fog and some urban pollution, aka urban ozone, block UV-B). The only way to know how much D you have and how much D or sun you need and if the supplemental D or sun, or tanning bed you are using is working is TESTING. TEST and RETEST, don't guess.
—KRISPIN SULLIVAN, noted vitamin D researcher, 2006

Vitamin D is found almost exclusively in animal/fish fats and not stored in any one organ.

The dogmas promoting low-fat diets, ultra-violet (UV) sunlight fear-mongering hysteria, and sun protection factor (SPF) sun-screen lotions have been responsible for rampant deficiencies of this life-saving nutrient (vitamin D) and its important co-factors. The body is able to manufacture vitamin D from a combination of its precursor ergocalciferol, vitamin D2, found in some plant foods, and cholesterol in skin when exposed to ultraviolet B (UVB) sunlight. Of course, this presupposes adequate levels of UVB sunlight (insufficient in more northern latitudes), adequate sun exposure (which almost no one gets even in sunny locations), and an absence of any sunscreens worn. SPF sun-screen lotions stop natural vitamin D production dead in its tracks and may actually make you *more* susceptible—not less—to various skin, and many other, cancers.

Living in the Pacific Northwest, where there are above-average rates of cancer and seasonal affective disorders, I have yet to measure D-levels in a person (other than yours truly) that showed actual blood levels even approaching optimal sufficiency.

If you have a need or interest in taking vitamin D, first take the time to get your blood tested. Anyone can order the 25(OH)D, or 25-hydroxy-D test online via www.directlabs.com without a prescription or a doctor's visit (blood can be drawn at any LabCorp location). It's relatively inexpensive. Keep in mind that standard lab ranges offered for comparison to your results, are ridiculously low, outdated, and relative only to everyone else who went into that particular lab system for blood work. Try, instead, to meet the requirements as laid out by the Vitamin D Council.

General blood chemistry caveat: These reference or lab-range values in *all* conventional blood chemistry reports are *not* standardized, or scientifically agreed upon, by anyone. This lack of convention is also true, by the way, of *every single blood marker* measured in standard blood tests—not just vitamin D.

As the population gets sicker and sicker and everything gets averaged out (with the useless exception of lipid panels, which are the only markers actually standardized, for the purpose of selling statin drugs) many lab ranges have become too broad to be meaningful to a major portion of the population. They don't tell you in the least how you compare with "normal and healthy." They are exclusively meant to reveal pathology, which may or may not be accurately represented. As such, many functional or sub-clinical dysregulations of, for instance, thyroid and other markers, go commonly unnoticed by your doctor. The American Endocrine Society and the American Association of Clinical Chemists both agree this is a significant problem. Scientifically standardized normal and healthy functional

---

ranges are available but typically used only by certain enlight-
ened natural healthcare providers (not all) and some Certified
Nutritional Therapists (CNTs), also referred to as Nutritional-
Therapy Practitioners (NTPs).

Far and away the safest manner of obtaining adequate vitamin D
is natural sunlight. In many areas of the country and during much of
the year, however, this can be an impractical (if not impossible) prop-
osition. Tanning beds using UVB bulbs can be another surprisingly
viable option. Vitamin D obtained via natural sunlight has no potential toxicity . . . though it *will increase your requirement for vitamin A.*
Note that only UVB will convert to D in combination with nutrient
precursors and cholesterol in your skin. If inclined to do so, always ask
for a tanning bed with the highest percentage of UVB bulbs for this
purpose, and patronize only reputable and sanitary tanning establish-
ments. Take care not to over-do it—a sunburn is never a good thing!

Make sure to take quality, high vitamin cod liver oil, too, to get
adequate vitamin A, especially after being out in the sun, as again,
sunlight exposure lowers vitamin A levels (Krispin Sullivan). Beta-
carotene and other carotenoids found in many vegetables and other
food sources may be additionally helpful to your skin as singlet oxygen free-radical scavengers and protective nutrients in their own right,
other than as a limited vitamin A precursor.

Those with diets excessively high in omega-6s (from soybean oil,
sunflower oil, canola oil, safflower oil, corn oil, and cottonseed oil),
trans fats and other processed fats, and excessively low in both saturated fat and cholesterol are far and away the most vulnerable to skin
cancers, as well as numerous other cancers.

Malignant melanoma, the deadliest form of skin cancer, has been
widely associated with vitamin D deficiency. *And what is everyone
rushing to do?* They lavishly apply sunscreens to supposedly prevent

the very thing for which they're actually increasing their risk. It's crazy! People almost seem to suffer from sunlight-avoidant hysteria. *The only people genuinely benefiting from sunscreens in this world are the ones who sell them.* Most SPF sunscreens utilize an omega-6 oil, likely rancid, type base, and tend to be formulated with many toxic and carcinogenic chemicals for the ultimate effect of blocking not only sunlight, but vitamin D as well.

Remember: the best protection against unwanted ultraviolet light is a good tan . . . or a hat. We evolved in fresh air and sunshine and have an actual nutrient requirement for sunlight—including ultra-violet light. Don't deny yourself your day in the sun!

We are designed, cell by cell, as creatures of the sun. Virtually every organ system in your body is dependent on sunshine for optimal performance. —AL SEARS, M.D. from *Your Best Health Under the Sun*

Vitamin D$_3$

MAKING THE
OMEGA-3 CONNECTION

Few are aware that omega-3 fatty acids—known also as alpha-linolenic acid, EPA and DHA—are easily the single most deficient nutrient in the modern Western diet. Insufficient intake of this vital and essential dietary component is linked with virtually every modern disease process, weight problem, affective disorder and learning disability.

Just what is omega-3, and what makes it so important?

Deep within the cellular structure (chloroplasts) of leafy green plants such as grass or plankton lies a substance known as alpha-linolenic acid, the "parent" form of a class of *essential fatty acids* known as omega-3s. The term *essential* means it cannot be manufactured by the body and *must* be supplied by the diet. When a grass-eating animal or plankton-eating fish comes along and consumes this substance in plant foods, a series of enzymatic and metabolic conversions take place to transform alpha-linolenic acid into its derivative forms: eicosapentanoic acid (EPA) and docosahexanoic acid (DHA). Herbivores make these conversions quite readily though are only able to make limited amounts of DHA. Humans make these conversions much less efficiently and numerous factors may complicate this process.

In order to initiate this important metabolic conversion, a critical enzyme, known as delta-6 desaturase (D6D), must be present. It is essential to the process of elongation and desaturation into the active derivative forms of omega-3 (EPA and DHA) from alpha-linolenic acid, found in green, leafy vegetable sources, walnuts and flax seeds. Once the body has either consumed or manufactured EPA, it can manufacture from this a series of eicosenoids such as series 3 prostaglandins, thromboxanes and leukotrines. All are essential to the functioning of the human body, as complex hormones functioning on the tissue or cellular-level.

DHA, another derivative, makes up the highest percentage of the fatty acids in the human brain, facilitating visual and cognitive function, forming neuroreceptors for neurotransmitters such as serotonin and dopamine, and serving as a storage molecule which the body may re-convert to EPA if needed later on. Omega-3s also make up a significant portion of all cellular membranes, giving them fluidity and helping facilitate all metabolic and bioelectric processes. No one can function optimally without them.

Although indispensable for the healthy functioning of the human brain and body, insufficient intake of omega-3 is a nearly unavoidable problem, endemic to modern diets, and can result in a complex array of symptoms readily contributing to our current national healthcare crisis.

Omega-3 (EPA/DHA) deficiency may be a contributing or causative factor in the following disorders:

- ADD/HD
- Dyslexia
- Depression
- Weight gain
- Heart disease
- Allergies
- Arthritis
- Violence
- Memory problems
- Cancer
- Eczema
- Inflammatory diseases
- Diabetes
- Dry skin
- Dandruff
- Postpartum depression
- Alcoholism
- Crohn's disease
- Irritable bowel syndrome
- Cirrhosis of the liver
- PMS
- Hypoglycemia
- Carbohydrate/sweet cravings
- Non-cancerous breast disease
- Ulcerative colitis
- Scleroderma
- Sjogren's syndrome
- Hypertension
- Bipolar disorder
- Irritability

- Soft or brittle nails
- Lowered immunity/frequent infections
- Frequent urination
- Fatigue
- Dry, unmanageable hair
- Hyperactivity
- Excessive thirst
- Dry eyes
- Poor wound healing
- Learning problems
- Alligator skin
- Patches of pale skin on cheeks
- Cracked skin on heels or fingertips

The metabolic pathways and conversions involved in the body's utilization of omega-6 and omega-3:

THE PROSTAGLANDIN PATHWAYS:
CONVERSION OF ESSENTIAL FATTY ACIDS TO PROSTAGLANDINS

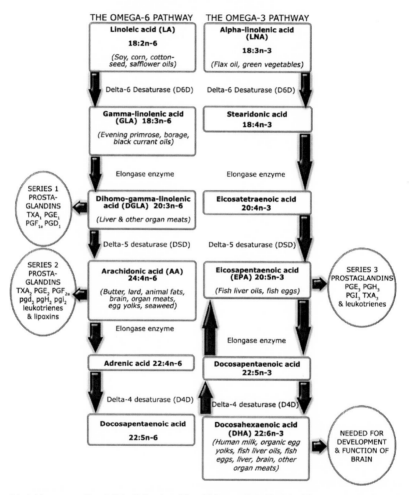

Adapted from source: Mary G. Enig, Ph.D., adapted from RR Brenner, Ph.D. *The Role of Fats in Human Nutrition* 1989

(Reproduced with permission from Sally Fallon.)

If we used to get so much omega-3, where did it all go?

Traditional/primitive sources of EPA and DHA in the diet have included such things as the meat and organs of wild game and other exclusively grass-fed meats and wild-caught seafood. At one time in our evolution, these essential fats were so prevalent in our diet it is hypothesized they alone were responsible for the three-fold increase in size of the human brain (Aiello, 1995). As much as 10% of human brain size has been lost in just the last century alone, likely due to decreased amounts of available dietary EPA and DHA and increased consumption of processed foods (Leonard, et al).

Increased consumption of grains and legumes—as well as nuts, particularly, seeds, and, more recently, vegetable oils—added excessive levels of another essential fatty acid: omega-6. Although omega-6 is needed in balanced quantity with omega-3 for optimal health, recent trends in agriculture, food processing and animal husbandry practices have resulted in dangerous dietary imbalances. As *delta-6* and *delta-5 desaturase* enzymes are needed for omega-6 metabolism, too, the resulting competition more often than not squeezes omega-3 out of the picture. The result is omega-6, including trans fats and others, dominates the composition of membrane phospholipids and those found in the brain and nervous system in the absence of much needed omega-3s. Excess omega-6—particularly in the presence of insulin—also results in excess production of *series 2 prostaglandins,* many of which promote and/or exacerbate inflammatory processes.

In today's world, however, excess omega-6 is not the only culprit interfering with *delta-6 desaturase* activity and utilization of omega-3. Among the most insidious sources of interference with this vital nutrient are man-made trans fatty acids, found in margarine, vegetable shortening, most commercial baked goods, nearly all fast foods, most processed foods, and commercial salad dressings and vegetable oils, including canola and soybean oils. They may appear on labels as "hydrogenated" or "partially hydrogenated."

Labeling laws do not require full disclosure of processing methods, however (due to certain loopholes in the law), and trans fat presence in most commercial vegetable oils remains largely hidden. Once consumed, it can take at least *two full years* for the body to get rid of dietary trans fats, causing untold metabolic chaos in the meantime (Enig, 2002).

Trans fats should be avoided *at all costs.*

Read all labels very carefully and avoid commercial canola and soybean oils, as well as all foods prepared with them (tortillas, potato chips, fries, boxed cookies, commercial breads, fast food, etc.).

Deficiencies of biotin, vitamin E, protein, zinc, magnesium, B12 and B6 all interfere with the action of delta-6 desaturase and other enzymes involved in healthy prostaglandin production. Consumption of sugar/starch also interferes with the desaturating enzymes and the concomitant production of excess insulin can readily divert omega-6 elongation toward pro-inflammatory prostaglandin pathways (Enig). As if all this weren't dismal enough, diabetes, poor pituitary function and low thyroid function are also synonymous with altered and inhibited D-6-D function.

Individuals of Northern European, Irish Coastal, Scandinavian, Inuit or Native American descent may not produce this enzyme at all and may actually have an increased requirement for EPA and DHA, due to the abundance of these substances in their ancestral diets. Deficiencies of omega-3 and insulin resistance are exceedingly common among these populations.

Sources

Modern dietary sources of omega-3 fatty acids, particularly pre-formed EPA and DHA, include wild-caught seafood from particularly cold waters, such as salmon, halibut, cod, herring, mackerel and sardines. Albacore tuna may contain small amounts. Farm-raised fish such as Atlantic salmon and other varieties are usually devoid of significant omega-3 content. Wild game is another excellent reliable source, though not everyone has access to this.

Exclusively grass-fed beef, lamb, venison and buffalo are also superb sources. Unfortunately, virtually all beef sold, even labeled "organic" in natural foods-type markets, *unless otherwise specifically labeled,* is feedlot-finished on grains, corn and soybeans, virtually eliminating all omega-3 content and containing highly imbalanced quantities of omega-6. Be warned, too, that all beef—even feedlot beef—spends at least part of its life out in the pasture and may be misleadingly labeled as "grass fed." Be sure to inquire whether *any* grain feeding took place prior to the animal going to market.

Web sites such as www.eatwild.com, www.grasslandbeef.com and www.grassfedorganics.com offer either regional or local sources and/or mail order sources for high quality, fully grass-fed and finished meat. Also, contacting your local chapter of the Weston A. Price Foundation can provide you with a wealth of local resources as well. (See www.WestonAPrice.org).

Regardless of whether one makes these healthy dietary changes, it is likely that, for a time, some period of additional supplementation of omega-3, EPA/DHA from either fish oil or Antarctic krill oil, may be necessary for remediation of deficiency states.

Supplements of flax seed and hemp oil are commonly promoted

rich sources of vegetarian omega-3s. Although this is true, flax and hemp oil contains omega-3 exclusively in its "parent" form, alpha-linolenic acid, and contains *zero* EPA/DHA. Alpha-linolenic acid requires the action of delta-6 desaturase and highly involved metabolic processes in order to be fully elongated and utilized by the body and brain in its most abundantly needed forms (see earlier detailed prostaglandin pathway illustration).

These conversions occur very inefficiently, if at all. Under optimal conditions and with certain individuals one might expect a maximum of about 6% of the alpha-linolenic acid in flax oil to convert to EPA and about 4% to DHA—assuming none of the aforementioned limitations are present. Should excess omega-6 and/or dietary trans fats be present, this percentage reduces to an average of only about 2.7% proper conversion overall, at best (Enig).

Clearly, flax oil is not the most preferable source of omega-3—particularly in a deficient individual—though there may be other benefits to flax oil supplementation and small amounts are okay. Walnuts also contain some ALA. Cod liver oil is an excellent source of omega-3 rich in EPA and DHA forms (also containing a little alpha-linolenic acid, as well), but it is mainly a vitamin A and D supplement.

Regular omega-3 fish oil or Antarctic krill oil supplements, combined with small amounts of cod liver oil, are far and away the best supplemental sources. Many companies molecularly distill their fish oil to remove any impurities or contaminants. Keep in mind that mercury is water soluble (generally concentrated in protein), not fat soluble, and is not considered a contaminant risk where fish oil is concerned.

Other very important adjuncts to omega-3 supplementation, include vitamin E, CoQ10 (when affordable), and selenium, which, in addition to vitamin D, protect these highly polyunsaturated oils from breaking down and going rancid. At the very least, some vitamin D and E should be added to any regimen using these highly polyunsaturated and delicate oils. The trace mineral selenium is required for vitamin E-complex (natural mixed tocopherols, rich in gamma tocopherol and preferably also containing tocotrienols) to work properly and is inexpensive to add to one's regimen. Selenomethionene is a highly bioavailable form of selenium and usually comes in 200 mcg dosages. Selenium may also be readily gotten from foods such as Brazil nuts, garlic and grass-fed butter.

Added fat-soluble antioxidant supplementation is critical with an elevated polyunsaturated fat, such as omega-3 or 6, intake. Also, dietary saturated fats, inherently resistant to oxidation, provide an important role in the protection and utilization of both omega-3 and 6. Unlike trans fats, they do not interfere with but actually help your body safely make the best use of these important and delicate nutrients (Enig).

It's never a good idea to totally avoid dietary saturated fats.

Dosages

Standard fish oil capsules contain roughly 180 mg of EPA and 120 mg of DHA. At these concentrations one therapeutic recommendation for remediating marked deficiency states of this nutrient involves taking one capsule for every ten pounds of body weight, preferably in two divided doses (Mercola). This translates to approximately one teaspoon of liquid-form omega-3 fish oil for every forty pounds of body weight (much easier). Another recommendation, offered by Dr. Andrew Stoll, MD, Director of the Psychopharmacology Research Laboratory and McLean Hospital Faculty at Harvard Medical School, is if you are using omega-3 fatty acids for health, mood or cognitive enhancement, roughly 2,000 mg/day is probably adequate.

Current research in the area of human longevity and life extension puts this at closer to 3,000 mg. Much is going to depend on how deficient and/or symptomatic you are. If needed for mood elevation or stabilization in more serious mood disorders or bipolar disorder, 10,000 mg of omega-3 or more may be appropriate. In these instances, capsules become far less practical, and using a liquid form makes more sense. The traditional Greenland Eskimo diet included at least 14,000 mg a day or more of omega-3. Where deficiencies are likely an issue as with ADHD or depression, it is probably better to err on the higher side, dosage-wise, for at least a period of time.

Always remember the increased need for fat soluble antioxidant protection with high dose omega-3 supplementation. EFA supplementation should at the very least, include added vitamins D and E with selenium. CoQ10 and R-Lipoic acid may serve some additional protection, if affordable. (*Note:* Anyone taking warfarin, or coumadin, high doses of aspirin, or any other related anti-clotting or blood-thinning medications should be under close supervision by their healthcare provider when combining them with high doses of omega-3 or vitamin E.)

If using cod liver oil, start with one to two teaspoons a day for children and one to two tablespoons or more for adults. Remember, our adult primitive ancestors probably received ten times the current RDA for vitamins A and D, and current research increasingly points to a greater need for vitamin D in the treatment or prevention of inflammatory disorders and cancer than ever previously suspected. Cod liver oil, a source also of omega-3's, in addition to vitamins' A and D is best used as an adjunct to other fish oil supplementation, particularly when therapeutic doses of omega-3 are needed.

A little flax oil added to salad dressings is okay—just don't try to use it as an exclusive omega-3 source—*and never, e-v-e-r cook with it!*

Efforts, particularly by vegans to compensate for low EPA or DHA conversion rates by increasing flax oil consumption proportionally can lead to a dangerously increased risk of stroke and cancer. Remember to always supplement with some preformed EPA and DHA and include some saturated fat and cholesterol in the diet for healthier, stronger membrane and vascular integrity.

Polyunsaturated vegetable oils have a weakening effect on cellular membranes in excess. Also, keep in mind that it is mostly rancid unsaturated and polyunsaturated oils lining clogged arteries and far less-so saturated fat or cholesterol. (Another myth bites the dust).

A newer source of EPA and DHA, Antarctic krill oil, may be a superb alternative for those who wish to avoid any fishy aftertaste sometimes present with conventional fish oils, and is also a source of an extremely potent, naturally occurring protective antioxidant or carotenoid known as *astaxanthin*. This, along with naturally occurring phospholipids, can actually improve utilization of EPA and DHA in the body and brain over conventional fish oil. Be prepared to pay big bucks for this alternative to fish oil, though—on the plus side, with Krill oil, "less does more."

Other important EFA considerations

Given the difficulty in relying on the activity—even the very presence—of the delta-6-desaturase (D-6 D) enzyme in the metabolic conversions of parent/vegetable forms of omega-3 AND omega-6 fatty acids to their active derivative forms, it is important to consider the plight of certain forms of omega-6 as well. D-6 D is also responsible for the conversion of alpha-linoleic acid (the parent form of omega-6) to gamma-linolenic acid (GLA), an important precursor to dihomog-amma-linolenic acid (DGLA), naturally abundant in liver and other organ meats. DGLA, in turn, gives rise to series-1 prostaglandins necessary for certain anti-inflammatory actions, as well as mood regulation, cognitive function, hormonal balance and prevention and treatment of skin disorders and may be conditionally essential.

It is probably advisable for most to consider supplementation with small amounts (recommended dosages on labels are probably sufficient for most) of either black currant seed or evening primrose oil to cover this base and prevent imbalances from occurring. Borage seed oil, although arguably the richest natural source of GLA, contains pyrrolizidine alkaloids that are known to be hepatotoxic. I'd avoid making this my sole source of GLA. Also, be certain these delicate seed oils are labeled as hexane and solvent free.

There are essentially three classes of prostaglandins. Prostaglandins are hormone-like substances made from essential fatty acids (EFAs) that operate on a cellular level to mitigate inflammation and various bodily processes. (Note: the process that gives rise to these substances, known as the prostaglandin pathway is outlined in the detailed illustration earlier in this chapter.)

Series-1 prostaglandins arise from GLA (gamma linolenic acid, a unique form of omega-6—found in evening primrose oil, borage seed oil and black currant seed oil) and DGLA (di-homo gamma linolenic acid, found in organ meats). Both have an anti-inflammatory effect

Series-2 prostaglandins are manufactured from arachidonic acid (AA), also an omega-6, commonly found also in organ meats, animal fat (especially pork), eggs, butter and seaweed. They are typically associated with pro-inflammatory processes (though this is a little overly simplistic). Both inflammatory and anti-inflammatory compounds may result from AA and this is partly mitigated by the presence of insulin

Series-3 prostaglandins are manufactured from omega-3s, more specifically, EPA, abundantly found in exclusively grass-fed meats, wild-caught cold water fish (such as salmon and sardines), as well in fish oil and krill oil supplements

Worthy of commentary here is the widespread controversy and vilification of arachidonic acid (AA), an important derivative form of omega-6 by popular writer Barry Sears, author of *The Zone Diet,* who insisted that this omega-6 fatty acid is to be avoided at all costs due to its pro-inflammatory properties.

Commonly found in liver, butter and eggs, arachadonic acid comprises 11% of the fatty acids found in the brain, is *absolutely required* for healthy cognitive functioning and is necessary for healthy inflammatory response following injury. There is also more recent evidence that the interaction of arachidonic acid with vitamins' A and D is absolutely essential for healthy neurotransmitter function. It is additionally the precursor to what are known as series-2 prostaglandins, some of which are inflammatory and some of which are anti-inflammatory. There are no "bad" prostaglandins—only imbalances.

Sears also asserts that perfect balance of the various prostaglandin series can be achieved by following a diet in which protein, carbohydrate and fat are maintained in certain strict proportions. This is a highly simplistic view of the complex interactions on the prostaglandin pathway, one which does not take into account individual requirements for macro and micro nutrients, nor of imbalances that may be caused by nutritional deficiencies, environmental stress or genetic defects. Like all systems in the body, the many eicosenoids work together in an array of loops and feedback mechanisms of infinite complexity. Furthermore, liver and eggs are both highly nutritious foods. Liver supplies DGLA, a precursor of the Series-1 prostaglandins, and both liver and eggs supply DHA, an important nutrient for the brain and nervous system. Arachadonic acid found in butter and eggs is also an important constituent of cell membranes(Enig).

Up to 20% of the population may actually be deficient in arachidonic acid. Furthermore, not all arachadonic acid derivatives are necessarily pro-inflammatory. Excess insulin from high carbohydrate diets, however, strongly influences the prostaglandin pathway toward inflammation and is ultimately the biggest culprit in chronic inflammatory disorders, especially when coupled with excess vegetable oil consumption. American diets are clearly slanted toward excess pro-inflammatory series-2 prostaglandin production in an unhealthy way. All prostaglandins, however, do have their rightful place in human physiology.

The optimal ratio of omega-3 to omega-6 fatty acids seems to be about 1:1, and no more than 1:4. Modern diets are supplying as much as twenty or more parts of omega-6 to every part omega-3. This invariably leads to undesirable consequences.

What is critical here is balance, not absolute amounts of any one type of fatty acid. Balance is achieved by observing three important things:

Adequate intake of viable omega-3 sources or supplements

Minimize or, better yet, eliminate dietary grains, legumes, feed-lot meats and vegetable oils (a little olive oil is okay), as well as other sources of sugary or starchy carbohydrate

Complete avoidance of trans fat sources, including margarine, vegetable shortening, commercially processed foods and baked goods, commercial canola and soybean oils, commercial salad dressings and fast food.

In the end, research seems to indicate that additional omega-3 supplementation over and above that needed to remediate deficiency states can be additionally beneficial to cognitive functioning. Inuit diets studied were shown to contain anywhere from fourteen to twenty or more grams, that's 14,000 to 20,000 mg, of omega-3, in combination with protective saturated fat, to no apparent detriment.

The bottom line here seems to be: If in doubt, it can't hurt to supplement!

"Your foods shall be your remedies, and your remedies shall be your foods"
—Hippocrates

THE TYRANNY OF TRANS FATS

Just what are trans fats, and why should we need to go out of our way to avoid them, anyway?

Trans fats are a form of artificially saturated, hydrogenated or partially hydrogenated fat typically made from vegetable oil (canola and soy are commonly used, though commercial lard is also usually hydrogenated). It is an involved, complex and exceedingly unnatural chemical process which takes largely polyunsaturated oil and combines nickel and hydrogen ions, along with a little bleach, coloring and steam-cleaning along the way, in an effort to change the chemical configuration into something resembling saturated fat.

Its commercial value lies in its ability to extend product shelf life. By altering this natural molecular structure, an "imposter" fat is produced that in no way behaves biochemically as its natural counterpart. Metabolic chaos is the result of trans fat consumption and the consequences range from neurological problems to cancer.

The following include some of the known adverse effects of trans fats in the human diet:

▶ Raises the atherogenic lipoprotein Lp(a) in humans
▶ Increases blood insulin levels in humans in response to glucose load, increasing risk for diabetes
▶ Decreases the response of the red blood cell to insulin
▶ Increases the risk of type II diabetes
▶ Lowers the volume of cream in milk from lactating

women, thus lowering the overall quality available to the infant

- ► Increased trans levels in human milk results in dose-response decreased visual acuity in breast-fed infants
- ► Correlates to low birth weight in human infants
- ► Decreased levels of testosterone and increases of abnormal sperm in males and interference with gestation in females
- ► Adversely interacts with conversion of plant omega-3 fatty acids to elongated omega-3 tissue fatty acids
- ► Escalates adverse effects of essential fatty acid deficiency
- ► Inhibits the function of membrane-related enzymes such as the delta-6 desaturase, resulting in decreased conversion of linoleic acid to arachidonic acid; alpha-linolenic acid to eicosapentaenoic acid (EPA) and docosahexaenoic acid (DHA)
- ► Causes alterations in the activities of the important enzyme system that metabolizes chemical carcinogens and drugs or medications, (i.e., the mixed function oxidase cytochromes P-448/450)
- ► Affects immune response by lowering efficiency of B-cell response and increasing proliferation of T cells
- ► Causes alterations in physiological properties of biological membranes including measurements of membrane transport and membrane fluidity
- ► Causes alterations in adipose cell size, cell number, lipid class, and fatty composition
- ► Increases peroxisomal activity (potentiates free-radical formation)
- ► A January 2001 paper in a peer-reviewed journal reports that margarine consumption is related to allergy in children, especially in boys

- Research reported in 1997 and 1999 showed trans-fatty intake related to asthma
- Dutch researchers reported in March 2001, that trans-fatty acids were again shown to be responsible for increase in heart disease and calculated that a 2% energy intake of trans-fatty acids is associated with an increased risk of heart disease of 25% *(The Lancet)*

(Above from Mary G. Enig, PhD, lecture at the National College of Naturopathic Medicine, October, 2001)

Because trans-fatty acids have no known health benefits and strong presumptive evidence suggests that they contribute markedly to the risk of developing CHD, the results published to date suggest that it would be prudent to lower the intake of trans-fatty acids in the American diet.
—NELSON, 1998 (G.J. Dietary fat, *trans* fatty acids, and risk of coronary heart disease. *Nutrition Reviews* 56:250-252; 1998)

The Danish Nutrition Council recommends that the addition of industrially produced trans-fatty acids to food stuffs ceases before 2005 and until then that the declaration of the content in foodstuffs becomes mandatory.
—STENDER, 2001

Clearly, hydrogenated and/or partially hydrogenated fats and oils have no place in the human diet. Obvious sources such as margarine, "spreads," vegetable shortening and products clearly labeled as containing "hydrogenated" or "partially-hydrogenated" oils are easy enough to identify and avoid. Few realize, however, that current labeling laws in the United States do not always require manufacturers to list the presence of hydrogenated or trans fats in foods and that their presence is far more ubiquitous than suspected. Virtually all pre-packaged snack foods, chips, cookies and baked goods contain hydrogenated or partially hydrogenated oils, often even when they claim to be "trans-fat free." They are able to get away from this because a certain amount of trans fat per serving is allowed before the manufacturer is required to disclose it on the label. All microwave-popping corn, for instance, contains partially hydrogenated oils, yet many claim to be "trans-fat free."

It's a simple, unscrupulous loophole—and far from harmless. Nearly all fast-food restaurants use these oils, and all commercial canola and soybean oils contain some levels of trans fats as a by-product of their deodorization process. Clearly, in this instance, reading labels carefully may not be enough.

Listed on the next table is the content of trans fats by weight percentage in several commercial bakery and snack-food brands and some typical trans-fat levels in U.S. foods:

Brands	# of products	Trans (wt%)
Bravo	1	49.7
Duncan Hines	1	36
Duncan Donuts	2	35.1
Entenmann	1	31.7
Frito Lay	6	25.8-47.4
Gerber	1	42.2
Giant	3	27.1-45.5
GNC	5	24.1-37.8
Keebler	4	29.4-46.9
Murray	4	33.1-35.2
Nabisco	14	12.6-53.9
Pepperidge Farms	14	10.4-28.0
Safeway	3	8.8-27.7
Sunshine	2	34.5-42.7
Thomas	2	30.4-32.5
Wise	2	15.4-36.8

*presented at the 1990 American Oil Chemists Society Meeting, Baltimore, MD
Data from Mary G. Enig, Phd, Enig Associates, Inc

A Quick Comparison of the Biological Effects of Saturated Fatty Acids vs. Trans-Fatty Acids, Just for the Heck of It:

1. Saturated fatty acids raise HDL cholesterol, the so-called good cholesterol, whereas the trans-fatty acids lower HDL cholesterol.

2. Saturated fatty acids lower the blood levels of the atherogenic lipoprotein(a), whereas trans-fatty acids raise the blood levels of lipoprotein(a).

3. Saturated fatty acids conserve the good omega-3 fatty acids, whereas trans-fatty acids cause the tissues to lose these omega-3 fatty acids.

4. Saturated fatty acids do not inhibit insulin binding, whereas trans-fatty acids do inhibit insulin binding.

5. Saturated fatty acids are the normal fatty acids made by the body that do not interfere with enzyme functions such as the delta-6 desaturase, whereas trans-fatty acids are not made by the body and interfere with many enzyme functions such as delta-6 desaturase.

6. Some saturated fatty acids are used by the body to fight viruses, bacteria and protozoa and they support the immune system, whereas trans-fatty acids interfere with the function of the immune system.

(from MARY G. ENIG, PhD—lecture at NCNM, October, 2001)

For countless years, scientists studying the effects of dietary fat lumped both saturated and trans fats together as being literally the same thing, making absolutely no delineation between the two. Nearly all research vilifying the biological effects of saturated fat have been greatly tainted by this and have been misleading consumers and healthcare experts for decades.

SO, HOW MUCH
NATURAL FAT DO I NEED, ANYWAY?

Current recommendations by the most knowledgeable lipid researchers and biochemists suggest an intake of *no more than* three to four parts of omega-6 fatty acids to one part omega-3 fatty acids. Omega-3 fatty acids should comprise at least 0.5% to 1.5% of the total daily energy, or caloric intake. Omega-6 fatty acids should comprise no more than 2–3% of the total daily energy or intake of calories. One-to-one ratios are probably more optimal. Higher intakes of omega-3 fatty acids may be desirable or necessary for a time (several months) to reverse a deficiency state.

Best sources of omega-3 include grass-fed or wild game meats and organ meats, cold-water, wild-caught fish such as salmon, herring, sardines and mackerel. Best supplemental sources include high quality fish and krill oils. Quality matters.

Please be aware: cod liver oil contains some omega-3 but is mainly a source of A and D. Raw, preferably soaked and dried, nuts and seeds are a rich source of parent form omega-6 oils and some parent form omega-3s. We do need some parent form, alpha-linolenic acid (ALA), found readily in fresh walnuts, flax oil and even in small amounts in fish oil supplements. Balanced omega-3 and 6 are also found abundantly in grass-fed meat and wild caught fish, along with needed protective saturates. Black currant seed oil and evening primrose oil are the best sources of supplemental gamma-linolenic acid (GLA), an important omega-6 derivative. Our ancestors got a lot of this, in the form of DGLA, eating organ meats. Periodic supplementation with these oils and/or increased dietary consumption of organ meats may be desirable in cases of GLA deficiency, due to impaired *delta-6 desaturase* activity, which manifests as eczema, skin disorders, hormonal imbalances, mood disorders and some forms of cognitive dysfunction.

Recent advances in leptin and life extension research point to a potentially important value in consuming a relatively higher *percentage* of fat in our diets (to be elaborated on later in this book). Implications of this research are very exciting and show how the very thing we thought was our worst enemy may well, in fact, be our best friend after all. Eating a diet containing higher percentages of dietary fat—using an optimized macronutrient ratio, and eating only as much as you really need to satisfy hunger—may actually help reverse disease and support radically increased healthy life spans . . . but we'll get to that.

What about ketosis?

Ketones are a perfectly normal constituent of human metabolism. They are used safely and effectively for energy in all tissues in the body, including the brain. In fact, ketones are *the* preferred fuel for every organ and tissue, and current research shows that they are a far less damaging source of energy than glucose, far more stabilizing, less excitatory and may, in fact, even help extend life span!

One particularly interesting study showed a marked benefit of a ketogenic diet for those with epilepsy. Children with epilepsy went on ketosis-inducing diets and their seizures essentially stopped (Prasad, et al, . "Alternative Epilepsy Therapies: the ketogenic diet, immunoglobulins and steroids." *Epilepsia* 1996; 37 suppl. 1: S81) The human heart prefers ketones, in fact, to any other fuel. Some evidence also shows that a state of healthy ketosis can help starve cancerous tumors, as they are unable to use ketones for fuel and must rely on glucose.

Vilification of ketosis was popularized by Jane Brody of the New York Times (a major proponent of low-fat, high carbohydrate diets), who warned of ketones as "toxic compounds." Dr. Luber Stryer, professor of biochemistry at Stanford University and the author of the biochemistry textbook used in most medical schools, says ketones are "normal fuels of respiration and are quantitatively important as sources of energy. Indeed, heart muscle, and the renal cortex use ketones in preference to glucose." Drs. Donald and Judith Voet, authors of another popular medical biochemistry textbook, say that ketones "serve as important metabolic fuels for many peripheral tissues, particularly heart and skeletal muscle." Far from poison.

Humans and hominids have been on ketogenic diets for close to the last three million years. Were ketones dangerous, it is unlikely we as a species would have survived to this day. In fact, both the body and brain actually prefer ketones as a fuel to glucose, as it is non-glycating and therefore non-damaging on a cellular level. Ketones are a steady, long burning, efficient fuel we were designed to use as our ongoing primary source of fuel for most things (except in an emergency . . . that's when glucose gets released as a turbo-charged supplement). We *always* pay a price for the use of glucose as an energy source, even in low amounts. Our red blood cells do need a certain amount glucose— it is unavoidable—but the less of it we use or depend upon, the better.

Having said the this, it is important to note that there are four instances in which a state of ketosis is potentially bad: for those with Type 1 Diabetes (ketoacidosis—a very different, more serious condition of particular concern under certain conditions—is sometimes confused with ketosis), those with renal disease, those who are pregnant (maybe), and those who sell diet drugs.

Ketosis is essentially the state where the body is burning fat for energy instead of carbohydrates. This is the state we all want to be in. Many ancient hunter-gatherers would have lived in a functionally ketogenic state most of the time. There is no evidence that it is a harmful state for normal healthy individuals to be in at all. To the contrary: the newest longevity and leptin research readily concludes that the more ketones you use for energy in your lifetime as opposed to glucose, the longer and healthier you will live—*by far*.

For those who are especially overweight and undertaking a more ketogenic diet, the initial excretion of ketones will be greater. During initial stages of weight loss in an individual who is insulin resistant, the body may be used to utilizing glucose as a more primary and inefficient energy source and may not yet be adept at utilizing ketones or burning fat efficiently. It takes time for the body to adapt to this change, and longer in older individuals than younger ones—about a month to six weeks for most, on average.

Care must be taken to drink a good deal of water so that more ketones may be lost through urine than the breath (which may impart an odor undesirable to some). This may also help dilute any toxic material commonly stored in adipose tissue that can get released in the bloodstream during ketotic states. *(Note: excess* ketones in the urine may be associated with diabetes and/or marked insulin resistance. This means you are excreting them, rather than burning them for fuel and are burning sugar, preferentially, instead. Some excess ketones are additionally passed in feces. Eventually—maintaining dietary consistency—the body adapts to the primary use of fat for fuel, and not sugar.

Utilizing additional herbal and antioxidant detoxification measures and supplements, which support improved insulin sensitivity, may be additionally beneficial in this process. Focusing on healthy and clean sources of fat in the diet is also important for these and many other reasons. If a person is not particularly overweight and is metabolically geared for burning fat instead of sugar, ketosis is a natural state and easily managed, if not entirely unnoticeable.

Supplementing with L-carnitine can also help minimize any discomfort, maximize energy levels during the initial stages of weight loss and help facilitate the transition to utilizing fat as a primary source of fuel. L-carnitine, which is not an amino acid but a quaternary ammonium compound that is a derivative of amino acid metabolism, assists in transporting fat into the mitochondria where it can be burned for energy. Supplemental pancreatic lipase may also help better facilitate the proper digestion and utilization of dietary fats.

In short, ketones are natural products of fat burning. When body fat is oxidized, ketones are produced. Unless you want to keep all the excess body fat you have, you can't and shouldn't prevent generating ketones. Period.

CARBOHYDRATE METABOLISM, 101

Annual refined sugar consumption in United States

1750:   4 lbs per person, per year

1850:   20 lbs per person, per year

1994:   120 lbs per person, per year

1996:   160 lbs per person, per year

Note: Global sugar consumption continues to increase by about 2% per annum, and in 2006–07 is expected to reach almost 154 million tons. *http://www.ers.usda.gov/Data/FoodConsumption/*

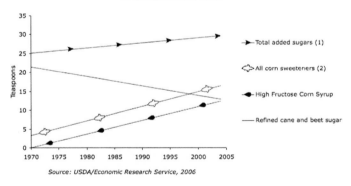

Added Sugar Consumption, 1970-2005
Average daily per capita teaspoons from the U.S. food supply, adjusted for spoilage and other waste

Source: USDA/Economic Research Service, 2006

All **non-fiber forms of carbohydrate** (from grains, rice potatoes and other starch-based foods), in addition to refined sugar, natural and industrial sweeteners (such as high fructose corn syrup) **are sugar, once metabolized by the body.** The dietary carbohydrate load in the human diet has grown unnaturally, exponentially and grotesquely from what our Paleolithic ancestors once knew. This includes starchy or complex forms, with the exception of indigestible forms such as fiber, as well as simple carbohydrates found in fruit. Wild fruit was a very different food from modern cultivated varieties (more tart than sweet, and very fibrous), and was only seasonally available, at best.

All non-fiber carbohydrates stimulate the secretion of insulin, the fat storage hormone, and/or damage the body and brain via a process known as glycation. Examples of carbohydrate foods in this context include: bread, pasta, cereal, rice, potatoes, granola, dried fruit, juices, candy, chocolate, desserts, alcoholic beverages, and even most fresh fruit.

Fructose, the simple sugar in fruit, may not impact insulin much, but it is extremely glycating, and damaging. In this context, the carbohydrates we are talking about here don't include fibrous vegetables and greens, which are very beneficial and have very little sugar or starch content.

The body is literally obsessed with maintaining glucose within a minimally necessary range, which may differ from person to person, depending on how dependent they have become upon glucose for energy and how insulin resistant they are.

There are actually several hormones designed to raise glucose, and only one that actually lowers it. This is because carbohydrates tend to be an extremely limited commodity in primitive diets and, as such, our ancestors very rarely had an "emergency" need to lower blood glucose, as is so common today. The ability to hormonally raise blood glucose in an emergency situation, however, is essential to survival.

It is fairly optimal for healthy, insulin and leptin-sensitive humans to have a blood glucose value in the bloodstream of no more than roughly 70–90 mg/dl at any given time (without any symptoms of hypoglycemia). Some current "functionally healthy" ranges are established as being more typically between 80–100 mg/dl, considered more the "norm," though lower ranges are by far more desirable for those who normally maintain low insulin levels, even if the higher range is more common in many individuals. Fasting blood sugar, from a functional standpoint, in excess of 100 mg/dl, is already reflective of dysregulation.

The state of hypoglycemia or even reactive hypoglycemia becomes a relative thing, depending on context. A fasting glucose level of 90 or 100 may feel like marked hypoglycemia and even induce seizures in someone who is used to levels of 400, as with some diabetics. Someone used to functioning between 80–100 mg/dl may feel reactively hypoglycemic (foggy, emotionally volatile or irritable) at 70. A healthy person maintaining consistently low glucose and insulin levels may not exceed 90 or 100 even following a meal and may feel absolutely comfortable and symptom-free with fasting blood sugar at 65. Again, it is relative and contextual.

The rule of thumb is, the lower you can maintain your blood glucose levels in a healthy and functional way (that is, without experiencing low blood sugar symptoms), the better off you are.

For those more optimally healthy, maintaining a range between 70–90 mg/dl or lower, this is equivalent to no more than 1 teaspoon of sugar, or about 5 grams, or 20 kcal, total. Keep in mind that the body is adamant about maintaining minimal necessary levels of glucose at any given time, as glucose is inherently damaging to vessels, organs and tissues in the body. The less glucose that is absolutely necessary, the better.

Two slices of bread, or a single small bagel, contain about 6 teaspoons of glucose—*five times* the amount normally allowed in the bloodstream! Dietary carbohydrates, with the exception of fiber are *all* absorbed by the liver and converted to the simple monosaccharide, glucose that is then released into the bloodstream. Cereals and potatoes can raise blood sugar even faster than candy bars!

Glucose in the bloodstream auto-oxidizes, which, in excess, produces potent free-radical activity, that damages arterial walls and forms cross-links with proteins called advanced glycosylation (also known as glycation) end products (AGEs). AGEs are known to accelerate the age-associated declines in the functioning of cells and tissues and cause mutations in DNA. AGEs bind with certain receptors in the bloodstream, appropriately called RAGEs, and induce widespread inflammation, leading to more advanced cardiovascular disease. A simple, inexpensive blood test that can measure up to a three-month window of glycation of red blood cells is called a Hemoglobin-A1C and can be used to more accurately monitor these glycation tendencies over time. Fasting blood sugar as a marker is not accurate for this.

Glucose is literally what ages (or AGEs) us. It is an irony that the very thing we all need to stay alive and fuel anaerobic processes is what science has discovered is ultimately what degenerates and kills us. We have to have *some* sugar to fuel our red blood cells, but not so much for our brains, as many think. Remember, our brain can run beautifully—in fact, better—with ketones, the energy units of fat.

Ketones are a much more steady, reliable and abundant source of fuel for our brains and organs to depend upon. Our red blood cells, however, need to burn sugar (glucose) for fuel anaerobically in order to preserve their precious cargo, which is oxygen . . . so they burn sugar instead of fats.

Unfortunately, in the end, we pay a price for what is somewhat inevitable. Aging is now being understood by those researching longevity as essentially a gradual process of tissue glycation of all tissues, including the brain. Chronic diseases associated with aging and certain forms of mental decline may be directly associated with these processes. The lower we maintain our blood sugar the slower this process occurs the longer and healthier we live . . . and the more gracefully we age.

A more pronounced and advanced state of the consequences of glycation effects may be seen in full-blown diabetics. The irony is that, given our most current understanding of how aging (which is now being viewed as a disease process) actually occurs, we can *all* be technically viewed as "diabetic"—to varying degrees.

Looking at it this way can really shift your perspective and hopefully your dietary habits. What is clear and irrefutable from current understanding of anti-aging medicine and how degenerative processes and DNA mutation (leading to cancer) develop is that the lower the levels of blood sugar one is able to maintain and the less insulin we produce, the longer and healthier we live and the "kinder" the aging process will be.

(*Note:* Glycation and its damage is ultimately a cumulative process, so every bit of sugar or starch we eat eventually counts. Every piece of candy, cookie, bread, potato, spoonful of honey or drop of soda drunk effectively shortens your life—something to think about. Though some glycation and/or its effects can be reversible, some are not. It's all a matter of what you choose to prioritize.)

Following a meal, significant levels of blood sugar generated above homeostasis stimulates the release of insulin that works rapidly to remove glucose from the blood. Whatever glucose is not needed immediately—for outrunning, say, a hungry lion via anaerobic energy (i.e., peak, turbo-charged energy output or exertion) converts rapidly to either glycogen, which is stored in very limited amounts in the liver and muscle tissue for times of extreme anaerobic exertion, or triglycerides—which moves into storage via lipoprotein lipase as adipose tissue (body fat).

We need to understand a certain rather major point: **our ancient**

ancestors never really had an emergency need to lower blood sugar. It's critical you understand this. And here's a news flash: Something even many doctors do not understand is that insulin's actual biological function and purpose is **not**, in fact, to regulate blood sugar. We have several other hormones actually designed for blood sugar regulation: glucagon, epinephrine, norepinephrine, cortisone and growth hormone. The regulation of blood sugar by these hormones is designed to *up-regulate* glucose when needed.

Insulin, by default, does lower blood sugar (very crudely), but insulin's primary purposes are actually to simply store away excess nutrients in case of a famine and regulate the coordination of energy stores with lifespan and reproduction. Blood sugar lowering is a trivial sideline for insulin, a key hormone that has much bigger fish to fry. This is hugely important to understand and a key factor in new understandings by scientists in the quest for advancing human longevity, which we'll cover later.

The need for steady fuel

Where "fueling the fire" of our brain and body metabolism is concerned, carbohydrates may best be described as "kindling." Whole grains and legumes are somewhat like "twigs" . . . starch, such as in cereals or potatoes, together with simple sugars are like "paper" on the fire . . . and alcohol might best be described as "gasoline" on the fire. If you're relying on carbohydrates as your primary source of fuel, you need to fuel that fire often, regularly and consistently. You will be craving that fuel. Unfortunately, most people today have forcibly adapted their bodies to such an unnatural dependence by over consuming carbohydrates in their diets.

Most if not all alcoholics (for instance) have severe issues with dysglycemia and sugar-addiction. Alcoholics are utterly dependent upon and regularly seek fast sources of sugar—alcohol being the fastest.

This is one reason why they say "once an alcoholic always an alcoholic." This is because the problem in alcoholism, in fact, isn't really alcohol, per se—but severe carbohydrate addiction. The typical AA meeting is replete with donuts, coffee and people standing around smoking cigarettes. Even though they may not be drinking alcohol, the damaging, often unconscious, sugar addiction in recovering alcoholics continues. Alcoholics are typically what I refer to as "carbovores", eating diets largely consisting of carbohydrate-rich foods, relentlessly craving sweets and additionally relying on stimulants such as caffeine and/or nicotine to constantly keep blood sugar levels up. The "sweet tooth" doesn't just go away with abstinence from beer, wine and liquor . . . hence the ongoing vulnerability to relapse. Once cravings for carbohydrates and the dependence on carbohydrates as the primary source of fuel are eliminated, so are the alcohol cravings. Training the body to depend upon ketones, rather than sugar for fuel is key to this equation. This essentially means eliminating sugar and starch from the diet entirely. Supplements such as L-glutamine can help the brain transition away from sugar in the meantime (sort of like "training wheels"), while the body adapts to its new, more stable and long sustaining source of fuel. Supplying additional nutrients that have been greatly depleted by alcohol and carbohydrate abuse is also essential to recovery.

One might get a burst or a ball of flame with respect to energy from many carbohydrate sources, but no one can get long-term, *sustainable* energy. As soon as the flame starts to die out, which doesn't take long, you're stuck with cravings for fuel or stimulants again. It can be quite a roller coaster ride.

This is why some dietary experts are always telling you to eat every two hours, or to eat "numerous small meals throughout the day." If you're sugar dependent—and almost everyone in this culture is victim to that unnecessary reality—then frequent small meals become necessary to maintain an even keel. Nature would never have intended for us to constantly live this way. It is a terribly impractical metabolic state to maintain, from the perspective of ongoing survival in a less certain world. Our primitive ancestors never would have made it this far.

Dietary fat, in the absence of carbohydrates, however, is like putting a nice big "log" on the fire. Fat's flame burns at a regular, even rate and is easily kept going. Protein, consumed in moderate quantities, is mainly diverted toward structural repair and maintenance. Only in excess does it convert to sugar. Fat's "even flame" keeps the hormone, leptin, under control, keeps insulin quiet, and keeps our appetites satisfied. Blood sugar—when one learns to depend on this steadier source of fuel—becomes a trivial concern. You become free to live your life instead of being constantly preoccupied with where your next meal or snack is coming from. One can go many long hours on this longer-burning type of fuel without experiencing any discomfort or cravings at all. You may eventually get hungry, if you really go a long time without eating, which is normal, but you are far less likely to experience irritability, dizziness, brain fog, cravings or mood swings because of it.

This is the way it's supposed to be!

What we have here is a failure to communicate . . .

Less than 1% of the pancreas is devoted to insulin production. Excessive demands for insulin can initially result in gradually reduced sensitivity of insulin receptors, leading to more and more insulin release needed to accomplish the same job.

This is what is termed "insulin resistance." In the earlier stages of pathogenesis of glucose dysregulation, a tendency toward hypoglycemia may be the result. Over time, however, the overtaxed pancreas may ultimately lose its ability to produce sufficient amounts of insulin, and type 2 diabetes becomes the problem. Once thought to be a disease of older adults, type 2 diabetes is increasingly becoming prevalent in young children.

In fact, diabetes is really not a "disease of blood sugar," but of insulin resistance—meaning the breakdown of communication between insulin and glucose. This is important to realize, as drugs which are designed to manage diabetes completely fail to address this issue and, instead, focus on lowering blood glucose, often using drugs that typically stimulate more storage of sugar as body fat. This does nothing to restore healthy cellular communication or reduce mortality from the disease. Diabetes drugs, though they may lower blood glucose initially, ultimately worsen the progression of the disease.

Obesity, in many ways, may be viewed as the price we pay for our body trying to stave off diabetes. In the end, however, the issue is one of communication breakdown and insulin resistance. *The key is the restoration of insulin sensitivity.*

So . . . how do we do that, you ask?

If you want to change the way any organization works, first, you have to go talk to the boss . . .

LEPTIN: THE LORD AND MASTER OF YOUR HORMONAL KINGDOM

Back in 1994, a discovery was made that shook medical science down to its core. They discovered a major hormone they didn't previously know even existed. Moreover, it wasn't just a major hormone; it was *the* major hormone which orchestrates and regulates all other hormones and controls virtually all functions of the hypothalamus in the brain. They found it in the last place they would have expected to: in our fat cells.

The name of the hormone is *leptin*.

Until the discovery of leptin, scientists believed that body fat was just an unwanted, ugly mass of excess, cumbersome energy storage. This view of fat has been changed forever. Body fat is now understood to be a complex, sophisticated endocrine organ.

A primary purpose of leptin is to coordinate the metabolic, endocrine and behavioral responses to starvation. It powerfully impacts our emotions, cravings and behavior. It turns out, in fact, that leptin isn't the only hormone secreted by adipocytes (fat cells) and that dozens of other hormones are produced there, as well. Many of them are pro-inflammatory in nature. In fact, leptin itself is an inflammatory cytokine and has a major role to play in the body's inflammatory processes as well. It also mediates the production of other inflammatory compounds in your body fat throughout your body.

Who knew the new kid on the block ran the whole neighborhood?

If you haven't heard of it, even if your doctor hasn't heard of it, don't be surprised. Drug companies have yet to create any drug that can positively influence leptin function, *Diet is the only thing that can do this.* (So much for fat pharmaceutical profits there.) Therefore, little about this important hormone is taught in medical schools or discussed in the media, despite its extreme importance. In all likelihood, you have either never heard about it or have only heard very little.

Leptin is a good hormone to get to know, though its function in the body is extremely complex. Understanding leptin is tantamount to understanding how to regulate the rest of your endocrine system, conquer your emotions, dramatically improve your health and even prolong your life. It's *the* single most important hormone in the body.

No other hormonal imbalance in the body, in fact, can ultimately be restored to healthy balance without leptin functioning normally. Keeping leptin levels healthfully low can prevent most diseases of aging and greatly extend normal healthy lifespan. High levels of leptin have been associated with most known degenerative diseases, inflammation, as well as obesity and a short lifespan. The more you can increase your brain and receptor sensitivity to this critical hormone, by far the healthier you will be.

Leptin essentially controls mammalian metabolism. Most people think that is the job of the thyroid . . . but leptin actually controls the thyroid which regulates the rate of metabolism. Leptin oversees all energy stores. Leptin decides whether to make us hungry and store more fat or whether to burn fat. Leptin orchestrates our inflammatory response and can even control sympathetic versus parasympathetic arousal in your nervous system. If any part of our endocrine system is awry, including our adrenals or sex hormones, you will never have a prayer of truly resolving those issues until you have brought your leptin under control.

This is a key thing to understand: the endocrine system is an exceedingly complex system of interrelationships that ultimately is regulated via an intricate hierarchical system of management.

At the top of the management pillar is leptin. Immediately below it is subservient insulin. Beneath that are your adrenal hormones, adrenaline and cortisol. Then, comes the pituitary hormones regulating thyroid and growth hormone (and others), then your thyroid, then your sex hormones . . . on down. It's a chain of command

There is not a single endocrinologist in the world, no matter how brilliant or talented—nor is there a single "bio-identical hormone" that can be prescribed—that could possibly replicate the intricate and delicate balance that is orchestrated by the interrelationships of your own innate endocrine symphony. Anything you do to micro-manage a single hormone in the body affects them all—and often in unpredictable and unanticipated ways.

Hormones, like a family, regulate together—and they dysregulate together!
—JANET LANG, D.C.

Hormones are measured in nanograms and picograms—billionths and trillionths of a gram! Hormones are not supplements (despite what "Dr." Suzanne Summers says). They are *extremely* powerful substances used in minute amounts in the body in extremely intricate and complex ways to manage your entire physiology. If you want to improve the functioning of your adrenals, thyroid or sex hormones, talk to leptin. Restoring healthy leptin functioning is the first major step toward ultimately restoring healthy endocrine balance, at any age, assuming your endocrine organs are intact and have not been destroyed or removed.

Just what dysregulates leptin and upsets your entire endocrine applecart?

The single most potent trigger of hormonal dysregulation is chronic carbohydrate consumption and subsequent blood sugar surges.

It turns out that leptin and insulin are birds-of-a-feather. The same things that tend to disrupt insulin also powerfully impact leptin. The worst offenders by far are dietary carbohydrates that are composed of either starch or sugar, and the blood sugar surges they produce—this includes bread, cereal, potatoes and other starchy vegetables, pasta, rice, and alcohol (yes, unfortunately, even wine and beer). "Natural" sugars, like honey, lo-han, agave, and maple syrup, as well as the refined versions, can all be similarly problematic. High fructose corn syrup is deadly. Medications of all kinds also contribute to leptin and insulin signaling problems. Caffeine and other stimulants similarly cause blood sugar to surge. The consumption of these substances, in turn, causes leptin to surge, which overwhelms the hypothalamus in a way that, over time, causes it to stop hearing leptin's messages.

The next casualty in line is your adrenals and what is called your "HPA" (hypothalamic-pituitary-adrenal) axis, which becomes dysregulated and may even additionally suppress thyroid function—effectively "turning down the idle" in an effort to preserve your "engine." The adrenals, constantly bombarded with the unnatural task of chronically regulating blood sugar extremes, become overburdened and may additionally "tune down" the thyroid to prevent total burnout during states of chronic stress.

That's where things start to unravel. The combination of leptin dysregulation, glycation, excess insulin, adrenal exhaustion and glucose oxidation are a "superhighway" to chronic fatigue, degeneration and disease. Toss in some trans fat to pound the last nail in the coffin.

> The only thing that can possibly restore healthy leptin functioning is a diet that is **very low in sugar and starch** (which includes eliminating grains, breads, pasta, rice and potatoes, as well as sweets) **and is sufficient in healthy natural fats.**

It's very simple and very cut-and-dried. Your Ice-Age primal body and mind are ruled by leptin. Adequate, not excessive, dietary fat—in the absence of dietary carbohydrates—is the optimal key to unlocking its power and potential to controlling your health, your well-being and your life span.

How do I know if I am "leptin resistant"?

Any, but not necessarily all, of the following symptoms can indicate that you are leptin resistant:

- Being overweight
- Fatigue after meals
- The presence of "love handles"
- High blood pressure
- Constantly craving "comfort foods"
- Feeling consistently anxious and/or stressed out
- Feeling hungry all the time or at odd hours of the night
- Having osteoporosis
- Unable to lose weight or keep weight off
- Regularly craving sugar or stimulants (like caffeine)
- Having high fasting triglycerides over 100 mg/dL—particularly when equal to, or exceeding, cholesterol levels
- A tendency to snack after meals
- Problems falling or staying asleep
- Your body seems to look the same, no matter how much you exercise

. . . Any of this sound familiar?

WEIGHT MANAGEMENT 101
AND THE PATH TO TYPE 2 DIABETES

Insulin is known as "the fat-storage hormone." It is regulated by leptin, though the same dietary influences impact insulin and leptin much the same way, and people can become resistant to the messages of both insulin and leptin in the same way. Again, they are birds of a feather. Carbohydrates such as sugar or starch are the primary dietary macronutrient that stimulates insulin release—as opposed to moderate dietary protein or fat—and generates unhealthy leptin surges which disrupt healthy communication and encourages hormonal resistance.

Ultimately, all body fat is made from glucose (*Basic Medical Biochemistry*). The hormone glucagon is required for the mobilization of fat stores and allows them to be burned for energy. Glucagon does not operate in the presence of insulin. If one consumes enough carbohydrate to stimulate insulin secretion, glucagon cannot function, and body fat cannot be burned.

Body fat cannot be burned as long as insulin is present. (Some things bear repeating!)

A fairly recent twelve-week study in Sweden compared the effects of a prehistoric (very low-carb) diet with what was termed a "Mediterranean diet" comprised of whole grain cereals, low-fat dairy products, fruit, vegetables and unsaturated fats. After twelve weeks, participants' blood sugar peaks dropped 26% with the prehistoric diet, and only 7% with the Mediterranean diet. (True Mediterranean diets actually look nothing like this.)

Again, diabetes is not a disease of blood sugar but of excess insulin. High blood sugar is a symptom of diabetes, but not the root cause. A diet excessively high in carbohydrates, which invokes excess insulin, leptin production and faulty hormonal signaling, is. Type 2 diabetics who are made to take insulin are actually ultimately worsening their condition over time, though they may experience temporary relief or "improved" blood sugar values. This is a deeply flawed approach. Elevated insulin and leptin levels are highly associated with, and even causative of, heart disease, peripheral vascular disease, stroke, high blood pressure, cancer, obesity and many other disease processes.

Since most treatments for (type-2, insulin resistant) diabetes utilize drugs which raise insulin or actual insulin injections itself, the tragic result is that typical, conventional medical treatment for diabetes contributes to the manifest side effects and the shortened lifespan that diabetics experience.
—RON ROSEDALE, MD

Dietary carbohydrate is at issue here, along with, to a degree, *excess* consumption of protein, which ultimately gets converted to sugar and gets stored via insulin as body fat. In fact, the more sugar-dependent metabolism you possess, the more readily your body converts other things, like protein, into sugar, too. In the end, fat cells are the last tissues to become resistant to insulin's messages. Becoming fat is your body's way of trying to delay the onset of diabetes.

A key point to understand is that **being fat doesn't come from eating fat; being fat comes from an *inability to burn fat,* which is a direct consequence of relying on carbohydrate—sugar—as a primary fuel source.**

Conversely, moderate protein consumption stimulates glucagon release and improves fat-burning efficiency via dietary-induced thermogenesis. It is important to note here, however, that *excess* protein in the diet will ultimately be converted to sugar and stored as fat in the same way. Remember—the more you over-eat carbohydrates and protein, the better your body gets at converting protein to sugar, *even if that protein is part of your own muscle and bones.* (Ever hear of osteoporosis?)

Most Americans do tend to over-consume protein, particularly from inferior sources. In the presence of excess carbohydrate, this is especially problematic, as the tendency toward glycation—damaging reactions between protein and sugar (Remember those dreaded advanced glycation end products, or AGEs?)—is greatly increased. Waste products from excess protein metabolism, together with the increased AGEs burden and damage our eliminative organs and capacities.

Baaad juju!

The downward spiral

As various tissues proceed to become insulin resistant, the liver—the first organ to lose insulin sensitivity and proper insulin signaling—becomes prone, as a consequence, to overproduce blood sugar from glycogen, which raises blood sugar levels even further. Eventually, other tissues lose sensitivity, also. Your fat cells are the last tissues to become insulin resistant. Your brain is unable to hear leptin's messages and your hypothalamus keeps sending you the signal to eat more, even when your fat stores are full. Your metabolism seeks to conserve fat in its state of perceived famine. Weight loss seems impossible. When your fat cells are finally no longer able to respond to insulin, there's no place for the sugar to go. It builds up in your bloodstream and you become diabetic, even if your insulin levels are still very high.

If it goes on long enough, you may even burn out your pancreas's ability to produce insulin anymore at all.

Other tissues unfortunate enough to lack the capacity for insulin resistance become chronically bombarded with excess tissue-damaging insulin and glucose. Among these, nerve cells are extremely vulnerable and become readily damaged by glycation, eventually developing neuropathy. Brain cells similarly are extremely vulnerable here, and deteriorate, rapidly glycate and oxidize, creating cognitive and memory problems and setting the stage for Alzheimer's. The arterial endothelium gets increasingly damaged and scarred by insulin and oxidation of glucose. Surges of insulin and leptin stimulate sympathetic (fight or flight) nervous system activity, causing the kidneys to dump magnesium and vessels to constrict, raising blood pressure and impairing cerebral and all vascular circulation. Vulnerable constricted blood vessels, clogged with glycated, oxidized plaques, and smaller vessels supplying the eyes and kidneys begin to become compromised, impairing blood supplies there. Vision and organs such as the kidneys may become impaired or seriously damaged.

In the end, you can be left blind, wind up on dialysis and have your limbs amputated. The risk of heart attack, all degenerative diseases, autoimmune disease and cancer is substantially elevated. It is not a pretty picture . . . and it is epidemic.

Hint: Osteoporosis isn't necessarily about low calcium

Again, a person predisposed to burning sugar as their primary source of fuel, particularly in diabetics, will have the tendency to more efficiently convert protein to sugar, also. Bones are largely composed of protein and collagen, which gives bones their strength and flexibility. Calcium gives bone their hardness. Hardness without strength and flexibility afforded by a protein matrix leads to weak, brittle bones.

If a "sugar burner" should attempt to starve themself or overly restrict calories, then the body will tend to convert its own protein stores from muscle and even bone to sugar to burn for fuel.

It's easier for your body to make sugar from protein than fat. This effect is also at play while asleep at night, where overnight blood sugar lowers, when you can't eat. This leads to a breakdown of vital tissues at night to support your sugar habit. These blood sugar lows, particularly in the presence of stressed out adrenal fatigue and depressed cortisol, also commonly stimulate nighttime catabolic (tissue breakdown) adrenaline releases, as the body desperately seeks to stimulate elevations in blood sugar. This leads to nighttime waking forms of insomnia and even middle-of-the-night cravings in some. Under extremes of stress, this can even result in muscle wasting, significant bone loss, immune dysfunction and possibly organ damage.

The loss of lean tissue mass in this way can contribute further to obesity and chronic fatigue, as the majority of mitochondria, our cells' own little energy producing "fat burning factories," are in our muscle. Inflammation, generated by excess omega-6, glycation, insulin, leptin, or anything else, readily destroys mitochondria. Carbohydrate consumption promotes inflammation. The less muscle and mitochondria you have, the less is your ability to burn fat and/or produce energy. With fewer and fewer mitochondria, you are sapped of your vital energy and can't lose weight. It is a vicious cycle. Even if you're thin, you're flabby.

The solution?

First, eliminate the sugar and starchy carbohydrates from your diet; this includes bread, pasta, rice, grains, beans, potatoes and all sweets and sweeteners. Limit fruit and stick mostly to berries when you do eat fruit (berries are lower in sugar, higher in fiber and richer in antioxidants than other sources of fruit). Second, consume just enough dietary protein to meet your immediate daily needs for rebuilding and regeneration from high quality, nutrient dense sources of *complete* protein, such as grass-fed meat, wild-caught fish and pastured eggs. This may be as little as 45–55 grams per day for most adult people (the approximate RDA), or just a few ounces—preferably in divided amounts (see the Protein Content of Foods Chart at the back of this book). Extremely large or active individuals, short of being an Olympic athlete, or individuals in a particularly nutritionally depleted state may need up to 10 grams or so more. That's really about all.

High protein diets are not advisable or necessary to be healthy and slim and can lead to numerous problems. The trick is in maximizing the quality of the source, digestibility of the protein—and/or quality of your digestion—and what you combine it with, so that you can make the best use of this precious commodity. This is not about inducing starvation in any way. In fact, if you go about it correctly, you should never be hungry. It's about improving the *efficiency* with which you use the quality, nutrient-dense foods in your diet.

Digestion takes more energy to perform than any other daily human activity. Eating more optimally sufficient amounts of *complete* protein—particularly when not overly cooked or combined with starches—actually greatly helps improve your digestion and assimilation of it, and you will expend much less energy doing so . . . which you will then have for other things! In fact, you may be utterly shocked to discover how much energy it is possible for you to have.

One of the other common causes of osteoporosis is poor digestion and/or nutrient deficiencies. This can include hydrochloric acid insufficiency (remember, HCl is needed to digest both protein and minerals, including calcium) and biliary (gallbladder) problems, leading to poor absorption of the fat soluble nutrients that are needed for absorption and utilization of minerals—particularly vitamins D and K. Taking vitamin D for healthy bones without also supplementing with vitamin K may, according to *the Nurse's Health Study*, actually double your risk of hip fracture! Roughly a dozen different nutrients or more are needed for the healthy formation of bone matrix. Eating a quality, nutrient-dense, whole food diet—and being able to properly digest it throughout life—is key to healthy, *quality* bone density

Hormonal imbalances in aging women, particularly inadequate progesterone, may also contribute to bone loss. Maintaining healthy adrenal function is essential for healthy female hormonal balance, particularly at menopause.

Finally, bone density has as much to do with physics as with chemistry. A sedentary lifestyle will result in significant bone loss over time. Weight-bearing exercise is needed to generate and maintain healthy bone density. Many people aren't aware that astronauts that spend time in space usually come back with significant bone loss . . . sometimes so severe that they are unable to stand or walk. The departure from the earth's gravitational pull causes bone to rapidly weaken.

Being a couch potato can have the same effect over time. Taking calcium pills is no more likely to build your bones than eating a side of beef is likely to make your muscles look like Arnold Scwartzeneger's. Bone develops (or shrinks) by the same principle that muscle does. Use it or lose it.

In a nutshell . . .

In sufficient amounts without added carbohydrate, dietary fat is satiating and calms the hormone leptin, which in turn helps control hunger and sends the message to the hypothalamus that "the hunting is good"—whereby fat stores become more expendable and more freely burned for energy. Fiber from vegetables and greens can be additionally filling, which may help, but it is dietary fat that actually satisfies the appetite, and prevents over-eating.

The more that dietary fat serves as your primary source of fuel and not carbohydrate, the better you will become at fat burning and the healthier, and naturally slimmer, you will ultimately be . . . **AND** the longer you will live. It turns out, in fact, that the very thing we have been told is our worst possible enemy actually may be our very best friend, if not our salvation. The idea here is not to eat a diet that is *excessive* in fat, but *sufficient enough* to meet the physiological demands for essential fatty acids and fat soluble nutrients, and satisfy the appetite. Using dietary fat in this way—while eliminating insulin-provoking carbs and moderating protein intake, as demonstrated by the very newest longevity research—is the deceptively simple and ultimate secret key to unlocking your health and longevity.

> **The key lies in minimizing calories while maximizing nutrient density.**

OVERCOMING WEIGHT LOSS MYTHS

Contrary to popular belief, healthy weight loss is not about increasing metabolism but about increasing the *efficiency* of metabolism. Why would you want the engine in your car to run hotter? People seeking to improve fitness and lose weight often exercise vigorously for prolonged periods of time in the hope that exercise will boost their metabolic rate. While this may burn calories slightly more rapidly, it also accelerates the production of dangerous free radicals. According to a prevailing theory of aging, oxidative damage at the level of the mitochondria is responsible for much of the inflammation and degeneration associated with aging (Heilbronn LK, de JL, Frisard MI, et al, 2006).

What you want is for the engine in your car to run more *efficiently*. Again, it's all about improving communication and signaling between cells and tissues via optimizing hormonal function, plus using the right type of fuel . . . and this is accomplished by minimizing the need for insulin and keeping leptin levels optimally low. This is best accomplished by eliminating sugar, starch and *excess* protein from the diet, and satisfying hunger by eating enough fat to satiate appetite—thereby teaching your body to burn fat rather than sugar for fuel—thus, maximizing your metabolic efficiency.

The idea that eating fat can help you lose fat may seem counterintuitive. It certainly conflicts with everything you hear or read in the media or get lectured about from your doctor or a conventional nutritionist or dietician. Yet, the most dramatically effective weight loss approach ever researched involved a diet that consisted of little more than 1000 calories a day divided into five, 200-calorie feedings every four hours, of *almost pure fat* (90%). Two British researchers, Gaston Pawan and Alan Kekwick, developed this diet after researching many different alternatives and macronutrient ratios. It has shown overwhelming superiority in burning body fat to even total fasting and no other weight loss regimen researched has ever come close to matching this diet's ability to burn off stored fat.

With no source of sugar to burn, the body is forced to burn fat. The adequate presence of dietary fat calms leptin levels and assures the hypothalamus that "hunting is at least okay," which keeps metabolism running efficiently. Caloric restriction then accelerates the weight loss. Of course, this particular approach is not a practical, advisable or long-term sustainable diet for anyone—it's woefully restrictive and lacks adequate protein and other nutrients—but the research underscores the impact of eating fat to burn even more fat than would be possible with a total fast.

Again, don't try this one at home, kids.

The point here is that eating fat—in the absence of carbohydrate—does, in fact, help burn more fat, and lots of it. You get good at anything by doing more of it. You don't get good at burning fat by constantly burning sugar.

For a more practical, sustainable and healthy version of this unwanted fat-loss approach the focus should be on nutrient-dense, animal-source foods, containing rich sources of natural, healthy fat and moderate protein. *Quality* **nutrient density is key here.** Adding bulk with sufficient quantities of fibrous, antioxidant-rich vegetables fills out most nutrient requirements nicely and staves off both deficiencies and hunger. Done correctly, this approach to diet actually maximizes your body's repair and regenerative potential, boosts your healthy immune function, allows for easy loss of unwanted weight and eliminates hunger.

"Most people mistakenly believe that low-fat diets are the only way to lose weight. They do not realize that the right fats, such as coconut oil and other healthy oils in synergistic combination, not only encourage weight loss but also help you heal. . . . "
—SALLY FALLON AND MARY ENIG, PhD from *Eat Fat, Lose Fat*

Fats and carbs together . . . a bad combo

The impact of dietary fat on insulin release is negligible, except in great excess or in the presence of dietary carbohydrate. When fats and sugar, or starch-based carbohydrate, are eaten together, the body will burn the sugar preferentially for fuel, storing more of the fat for later.

Sugar is such a damaging substance to the body that the body will race to rid itself of excesses as quickly as it can. The body does this first by rushing as much sugar as possible to cells with the help of insulin as a means of producing immediate, anaerobic, turbo-charged energy—the equivalent of putting rocket fuel in your car. If this is not immediately needed (in other words, if you don't happen to be trying to outrun a charging rhino), then much of the sugar is converted first to glycogen and stored in the liver and muscle tissue. Once this very limited capacity for storage is filled, your body proceeds to convert what is left to triglycerides in the liver, and stores whatever is left in your fat cells.

If one is insulin resistant, energy or glucose can't get into cells for fuel and must be converted to fat and stored for another time. This is all a very inefficient and energy-intensive process that tends to generate fatigue or sleepiness after meals as a person gradually becomes insulin and leptin resistant. In this state, you are basically unable to make use of the energy in your food. Dietary fat that isn't otherwise utilized elsewhere in the body and can't get burned for energy is first converted to sugar, then re-converted to triglycerides for fat storage—a complex and energy intensive process.

Next . . .

By increasing the amount of stored body fat, leptin levels automatically rise. With elevated leptin, an inflammatory cytokine, inflammation increases throughout the body. This is one major reason overweight and obese people are so at risk for degenerative illness, heart disease and cancer—raging chronic systemic inflammation. Furthermore, these surges of insulin and leptin increase sympathetic over-arousal, anxiety and stress hormones. (Know anyone with chronic anxiety or trouble sleeping?)

Elevated stress hormones, when being produced in such a damaging cycle, catabolize or break down tissue as well as weaken our immune system. A protective substance lining our GI tract known as *secretory IgA*—the first defense in our immune system—is broken down under chronically high (**or** excessively low, as occurs in adrenal burnout) cortisol levels. This leaves the small intestine vulnerable to something known as "leaky gut syndrome." This is where undigested proteins and other substances that normally are not allowed across the semi-permeable intestinal barrier are able to get across and trigger antibody responses that may either elicit allergic, or physical, emotional or cognitive sensitivity reactions. As the vicious cycle continues and cortisol/adrenaline/insulin/leptin levels climb, what is known as "TH2" (T-Helper cell 2) antibody immune response can up-regulate, and the "TH1" (T-Helper cell 1) humoral immune response can down-regulate, leading to more exaggerated food sensitivities, as well as others. The suppression of TH1 leaves one more vulnerable to contagions and illness or infection (Know anyone who gets colds all the time and has allergies or food sensitivities?). This cycle can be very difficult to bring under control and tends to be self-perpetuating. Food sensitivities add unwanted cortisol and insulin levels and can be a very common source of weight gain for some.

The excesses of fat, being generated by insulin and cortisol, also more readily secrete enzymes that stimulate the excessive conversion of testosterone to estrogen in men—the #1 cause of seeming testosterone deficiency in men, in fact—and the conversion of estrogen to toxic DHT testosterone in women, making weight-loss extremely difficult.

This can make one appear testosterone or estrogen "deficient" in blood or salivary tests. Lower testosterone levels also make men more prone to dopamine neurotransmitter deficiencies, as depressed testosterone also depresses dopamine receptor activity. Excessively lower estrogen levels in women suppress serotonin receptor activity and increase proneness to depression and other issues.

The answer here is almost never "hormone replacement"—even with "bio-identical" hormones, which only temporarily alleviate the symptoms and can eventually greatly exacerbate the problem. You may feel temporarily better with supplemental estrogen, or even feel like superman, at least for a while, on the supplemental testosterone . . . but in the end, you are only making the problem worse. The underlying answer is in controlling this whole cascade of events by basically doing what is necessary to manage leptin, insulin and your adrenals. The excessive conversion of hormones is an extremely vicious cycle and is at the heart of what is known as "syndrome X" or "metabolic syndrome."

It cannot be "micro-managed" by hormone replacement.

Why calorie counting doesn't work

It seems everyone who wants to lose weight becomes fixated on one common pass-time: "counting calories." It becomes an obsession for some. The whole principle behind the concept of dietary calories lies in the potential of a given food to generate energy or heat. Using this as a measure of which food should and shouldn't be eaten presupposes, however, that the human body is mainly a "heat engine" and solely consumes food for the purpose of producing energy or heat.

This simply isn't so and makes for a deeply flawed approach, destined for bigger problems.

The human body is, in fact, a complex "chemical factory." Different food substances are eaten, utilized and processed in many different ways, and the utilization of different macronutrients is far from equal. Energy is far from the only thing extracted from what we eat. Protein, for instance, largely goes to building, rebuilding or maintaining structure in the body, including skin, bones, hair, lean tissue, hormones, neurotransmitters and innumerable other cellular components. It is estimated that the human body manufactures over 50,000 different proteins in various forms for ongoing processes and structure. In the case of dietary protein, it is only excess amounts that get converted to sugar and stored as body fat or unwanted calories.

Since we are fairly efficient at recycling our protein stores, only a few ounces of concentrated, complete protein per day are actually *needed* by all but the most active or depleted individuals. The problem with trying to meet protein needs with vegan sources of protein lies in the incomplete amino acid profile and/or the high starch content of nearly all "vegan-source" protein-containing foods. Without having four stomachs, or an herbivore's metabolic system, we're just not designed to pull it off. Even trying to combine proteins to obtain a complete amino acid profile ends up usually lacking in actual protein sufficiency (even with our minimal needs). A vegetarian or vegan-based diet is always ultimately a starch-based diet . . . and we're not cows—we can't just do it all with veggies long term. *We need the nutrient density.*

But I digress.

Dietary fats also have a complex, profound and varied role to play in physical structure and function. Dietary fat—arguably the most important macronutrient, with the possible exception of water—primarily serves the needs of innumerable physiological processes: building, rebuilding and maintaining cellular membranes and nerve tissue; manufacturing hormones and neurotransmitters; facilitating cellular communication and absorption of fat-soluble nutrients; stabilizing the nervous system, supporting the immune and lymphatic systems; creating pro- and anti-inflammatory compounds; supporting proper utilization of proteins; as well as fueling the brain, heart, and other muscles. (Whew!)

Most fat gets absorbed, not into the bloodstream but into the lymphatic system. Again, only excess fat gets converted first to sugar, then to body fat for storage—a very energy inefficient process. Certain shorter chain fats, however, such as those found in butter (butyric acid) and especially coconut oil (medium chain triglycerides, or MCTs) have potent antimicrobial activity, are similar in caloric value to carbohydrates, are nearly always burned preferentially for energy and do not easily store as body fat. These short and medium-chain fats may, in fact, help energize and fuel weight loss!

Carbohydrates, on the other hand, have a minimal role to play as any sort of structural compound in the body. Less than about 2% of bodily structure is composed of carbohydrate, and *all* of this can be manufactured without the presence of dietary carbohydrate. Certain *glyconutrients* serve as components of joint tissue and cartilage. Certain other glyconutrients play a unique role in immune function. Fiber—a "non-utilizable carbohydrate"—essentially serves as bulk in the diet and may help facilitate waste elimination in the colon (though is not essential for that) as well as serving to bind excess conjugated hormones and allow for their proper excretion. Apart from this, the body uses only minute amounts of sugar to fuel red blood cells and is able to store all of about 2,000 calories worth as glycogen in the liver and muscles for emergency use for major exertion. *All the rest*—every single calorie of carbohydrate consumed that is not immediately required for turbocharged, anaerobic effort—is converted in a limited way to glycogen, then the rest to triglycerides by the liver and stored as body fat . . . at least, as long as insulin is willing to keep facilitating the effort.

Once one is insulin resistant from constant bombardment of dietary carbohydrate, for which there is a *zero* dietary requirement, sugar simply begins to build in the bloodstream. There, it accelerates glycation of red blood cells and endothelial tissue, forming advanced glycation/glycosilation endproducts (AGEs), generating increased free radicals, untold oxidative damage and rampant systemic inflammation. The body undergoes activation of genes that up-regulate certain enzymes to better facilitate burning of sugar as a primary source of fuel (an unnatural prolonged metabolic state), in an effort to just to get rid of it. *And fat burning comes to a screeching halt.*

You are one of two things: you are either a "fat burner" or a "sugar burner." If you are overweight, crave carbohydrates (and stimulants) or are leptin-resistant, then you are a "sugar burner."

It also should be noted that stress, food sensitivity issues, caffeine or stimulants, alcohol, sleep deprivation, aspartame, tobacco and drugs of all types further aggravate and exacerbate excess insulin production (Schwarzbein, 1999).

For those who are unconcerned about dietary carbohydrate from a weight-gain perspective due to higher metabolism levels or athletic activity, the caution is this: *Although it is possible to burn off the excess glucose, one cannot "burn off" the excess insulin.* Excess insulin production, no matter how thin you are, wreaks metabolic havoc and invariably yields unhealthy consequences over time and accelerates aging.

It is also possible to be thin and diabetic.

THE HIDDEN (AND NOT-SO-HIDDEN) RAVAGES OF BLOOD SUGAR DYSREGULATION

Glucose dysregulation and excess dietary carbohydrate can ultimately manifest as a vast array of disorders including, but not limited to:

- Frequent illness/immune disorders
- Serotonin depletion
- Candidiasis
- Fatigue
- Dizziness
- Irritability
- Depression
- Anxiety
- Confusion and memory problems
- Night sweats
- Weight problems
- Alcoholism
- Nervous habits
- Mental disturbances
- Insomnia
- Heart disease
- Adrenal insufficiency
- Thyroid disorders
- Pituitary disorders
- Kidney disease
- Pancreatitis
- Chronic liver failure
- Diabetes/Hypoglycemia
- Cancer

Among the simplest telltale signs of insulin and leptin resistance are the appearance of "love handles," and/or cravings for either carbohydrates or sweets, or stimulants (such as caffeine) and/or sleepiness or fatigue after meals.

Ensuring quality moderate dietary protein and omega-3s in the diet, along with reducing sugar and starchy carbohydrate, vegetable oils and margarine consumption, can help restore insulin sensitivity and reduce or eliminate many associated symptoms of insulin resistance or glucose dysregulation. Also important is *limiting or eliminating the use of caffeine and other stimulants, alcohol, tobacco, artificial sweeteners, all recreational drugs and unnecessary over-the-counter and/or prescriptive medications* (Schwarzbein, 1999).

Engaging in stress-reduction activities and exercise helps further. Numerous supplements may also help accelerate improved insulin function. Over time, insulin sensitivity may be restored through careful attention to these important dietary principles, some appropriate supplementation and a reduced-stress lifestyle.

BUT WHAT ABOUT EXERCISE?
WON'T THAT MAKE UP FOR IT?

In a word, no.

Exercise is certainly "something-better-than-nothing" toward helping the situation. It can *help* in restoring insulin sensitivity and burn off some excess carbohydrate and fat, depending on the type of exercise done—but not all exercise is created equal nor is necessarily always beneficial. If you are a "carbovore," however, you may never get around to effectively burning your fat stores.

Exercise can never compensate for a lousy diet—any more than drugs or supplements can. At least 70% or more of your health equation resides in diet. Most of the other 30% is a combination of appropriate supplementation, stress reduction, positive attitude and exercise. Exercise is a helpful component of healthy weight loss in tandem with a healthier diet. The key is the *quality* and not a high quantity of exercise.

Although the details of this topic are best saved for a separate book, suffice it to say that brief bouts of peak, anaerobic exertion are essentially superior to expanding the health of the heart and lungs and in facilitating weight loss and/or lean tissue development. More exercise is not better, contrary to the common tendency of those who endeavor to jog endlessly on their treadmills or spend hours in the gym lifting weights.

Our ancestors never would have bothered with such wasteful and wearing expenditures of energy! Consider that, apart from walking, "exercise" for our Paleolithic ancestors mainly consisted of brief bouts of running to catch things they were hunting, or running away from things that wanted to eat or trample them. These brief, intense bouts of exercise served to expand heart and lung capacity, challenged and developed the strength of skeletal muscles, and rapidly used blood glucose and glycogen stores. Now, you might be thinking "That doesn't burn any fat!"

Au contraire.

Consider what message you send your body when you spend hours jogging on a treadmill. After about the first twenty minutes of exercise, when the body changes over from predominant use of glucose to predominant use of body fat, we go into that "fat-burning mode" that aerobic exercise pundits tell you is "the zone." But what is this really telling the body when we spend extended amounts of time in this so-called "zone"? It is saying, "Hey, we're being asked to do this ridiculously tedious and demanding thing and it's going to require *a lot of fat.*"

Make no mistake about it, you *will* burn some fat doing this . . . but remember that fat to our physiology means survival, and if it's going to take a lot of that precious commodity to fuel what we're doing, our body is going to work at becoming more efficient at making this fuel available. It will become better at converting everything you eat into fat and burn more efficiently and sparingly over time so it becomes harder to use it up. God forbid you should fall off your exercise wagon. You will rapidly gain back whatever you may have lost (and then some) while your body's energy stores prepare for the next marathon. (Yes—fat is a vastly better, more efficient and long-lasting fuel for marathons than carbohydrates. "Carb loading" for marathons is more than a myth—it's a big, big mistake. This was proven conclusively in studies done at the University of Buffalo, New York.)

All the while you're plodding along on your treadmill, you are also effectively telling your heart and lungs they don't have to be any stronger or more capable than what you're asking them to do. You will actually *lose* cardio-pulmonary capacity over time, even weakening your heart. (Remember Jim Fixx, the founder of the jogging craze who dropped dead of a heart attack?) Furthermore, exercise is a form of stress on the body. We can tolerate—and are well designed to tolerate—*brief* bouts of peak effort, from which our adrenals require a certain amount of time, a good 24 hours, to fully recover. Our body strengthens in response to peak effort in a way that makes us stronger and faster the next time. That's the way we were designed.

But what happens when we pound or lift away, unnaturally for long exercise periods in the gym? We produce a lot of cortisol, our primary stress hormone . . . and cortisol, in turn. both raises blood sugar and is *catabolic* in nature. In other words, *cortisol eats muscle and other tissues for lunch.* (Remember, too, that your heart is also a muscle.)

You are making one sweaty step forward and two, big, wasted (or worse) steps back. Chronic cortisol production suppresses the immune system and breaks down your muscles as fast as you're trying to build them. The elevations in blood sugar stimulated by cortisol also stimulates more insulin—not a desirable thing for improving insulin sensitivity or healthy blood sugar—and little of positive value is accomplished.

Furthermore, once you've finished your extended bout of "aerobic" exercise, the fat burning more or less stops, or substantially slows there. This is an extremely inefficient means of losing body fat.

With brief, intense anaerobic training however, there is a residual fat-burning effect that can last up to *two days!* There is an "after effect" known as excess post-exercise oxygen consumption, or EPOC, which in effect ramps up the weight loss for extended periods of time—even while you're sleeping! A scientific study that was done by

Laval University proved that short, intense workouts burn up to **nine times more fat** than traditional aerobic training.

So ... what do you do?

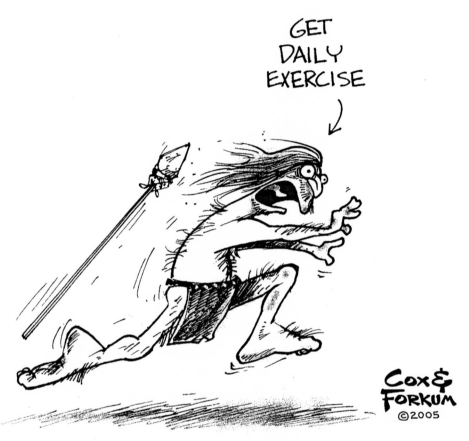

www.CoxAndForkum.com

First, limit exercise to no more than fifteen to twenty minutes in duration, and focus on brief bouts of significant *anaerobic exertion,* interspersed with brief periods of recovery at a slower pace sufficient for returning to resting heart rate. This may be done via sprinting, cycling, rowing, elliptical machines ... whatever. Or, it may be done using weights or calisthenics, where muscles are, after warming up, challenged close to their peak capacity for a set or two. Strength or resistance training reverses the reduction in muscle fiber size that accompanies aging and inactivity and has been shown conclusively to increase insulin sensitivity. Study after study has shown that resistance training is superior to aerobic exercise in improving insulin receptor sensitivity—and even aerobic capacity! It also lowers insulin levels.

Once each muscle group has had its neural recruitment capacity sufficiently challenged and has performed its peak exertion, you are done for the day. This may take no more than 10–15 minutes, total. Another way of going about it can be "sprinting" (biking, rowing, swimming, elliptical training, etc.) for four or five sets of up to a minute each, allowing for heart rate recovery in between. This exercises and expands heart and pulmonary capacity, as well as honing strength. Talk about a time and life saver!

Done appropriately, this can be adopted by anyone, regardless of his or her age or fitness level, with or without a gym. Changing your routine and type of exercise daily is another means of enhancing your gains and eliminating plateaus. Don't let your body get too used to any one routine. Also, working muscles in "groups," or "whole body" exercises, rather than as "a collection of individual body parts" using isolation exercises or machines is infinitely more efficient, effective and natural. Following this, critical building and rebuilding mechanisms can immediately take place over the next day or two to make you ultimately better and stronger than you were before.

This is how evolution designed us to achieve fitness—not by running marathons or standing around doing arm curls.

In exercising for brief, intense bouts, you become more readily efficient at storing future sources of carbohydrate as glycogen in muscle—increasing the size and definition of the muscle and better fueling it in the future—instead of simply converting it to body fat to fuel the marathons. You better preserve your precious adrenal health. Enhanced muscle growth, stimulated by growth hormone during peak effort, increases the number of mitochondria in the body—our body's little fat-burning factories, found almost exclusively in muscle—and thus, inherently enhances our use of fat as fuel and consequently our energy, as well. This also ensures that your body more comfortably releases fat stores for fuel, since no undue demands are being placed upon endurance capacity. You become a lean, mean, fat-burning machine!

For additional information regarding this general approach to cardio-fitness and/or body building or strength training, get Dr. Al Sears' book, *PACE* (for "Progressive Accelerated Cardiopulmonary Exertion") for advanced, excellent and possibly the best detailed education on the subject (2006). You can also visit the web site: http://www.alsearsmd.com/pace/. For other related reading and additionally effective approaches that are compatible, Lawrence E. Morehouse, PhD, and Leonard Gross's book *Maximum Performance* is excellent (1977). For those interested mainly in body building, read anything by Mike Mentzer; and for general fitness and strength training, Pavel Tsatsouline (former physical training instructor for the Soviet Special Forces, author, and no-nonsense fitness training expert). Tsatsouline also has several DVDs.

For those not in need of weight loss who just want to develop their strength and flexibility, yoga and other core strengthening exercises may be useful. Some anaerobic training for improving cardio-pulmonary capacity is *always* a good idea, though.

Increased lung capacity, more than any other single physical factor, is tantamount to greater longevity.

THINGS THAT MAY HELP
CONQUER SUGAR CRAVINGS,
MINIMIZE OR HELP REVERSE GLYCATION
AND RESTORE INSULIN SENSITIVITY

*N*ote: It is not necessarily suggested that you need to take all the supplements presented below. This is merely a guide to many known to be additionally helpful to the basic dietary guidelines presented.

▶ Eliminate sugars and starches from the diet. (*Note:* if you are extremely insulin resistant or diabetic, it may be a more gradual process of converting metabolically to the use of fat as a primary source of fuel and may best be facilitated and accomplished in tandem with additional supportive supplements)

▶ Consume moderate amounts of nutrient-dense protein and enough natural dietary fat to satisfy hunger. This greatly helps normalize blood sugar levels. Be sure to get adequate essential fatty acids, particularly EPA, DHA and GLA

▶ Regularly take a B complex (preferably phosphorylated, food complexed or co-enzymated) with meals. B vitamins assist in improved carbohydrate metabolism. Vitamin B-1 and especially its fat-soluble derivatives, allithiamine, or *benfotiamine.* (100–250 mg or more, if needed), can greatly help reduce glycation.

▶ L-carnosine is an amino acid that may serve as a powerful neuroprotective, anti-glycating nutrient. Take 500–1000 mg, one to two times daily

- L-carnitine (not to be confused with L-carnosine) is a quaternary ammonium compound and an amino acid derivative, not an actual amino acid, necessary for transporting fatty acids into the mitochondria where they can be burned for energy. It can reduce the time it takes to convert from "sugar burning" to "fat burning" in resistant individuals. (2,000 mg or more/day)
- Acetyl-L-carnitine is fat-soluble and is better able to protect and aid in fueling the brain than regular L-carnitine. It is ultimately anti-glycating and, especially in tandem with R-Lipoic acid, has been shown to markedly reverse neuropathy. (500–2000 mg/day)
- Supplemental chromium—chromium is a trace mineral essential to normalization of glucose metabolism. 200–400 mcg per day of chromium picolinate or GTF chromium is usually sufficient
- R-Lipoic acid—this functions as an antioxidant—is uniquely effective against both fat-soluble and water-soluble free radicals, can prevent and even help reverse glycation, improve blood sugar metabolism and improve cellular energy production. (50–250 mg/day) . . . More may be needed by some.
- Benfotiamine—a powerful, fat soluble version of vitamin B1 that is known to significantly inhibit the formation of AGEs and help prevent damage to nerves and small blood vessels caused by glucose. Its fat solubility also gives it better overall bioavailability and passage to the interior of the cell where it can prevent glycation within the cell, where our vulnerable DNA lies. (100–250 mg/day has been used in studies, with often dramatically positive effect)
- Pyridoxamine—a unique form of vitamin B6 that specifically interferes with toxic glycation reactions. May be the most potent natural substance for inhibiting AGE formation. (50–100 mg commonly used in studies reporting beneficial effects.)
- Trans-resveratrol—originally found in grape skins and red wine, this compound has shown itself to have many dramatic and

exciting potential benefits to health . . . among them significantly improved insulin sensitivity. The down-side is its exorbitant cost. Recommendations include taking no less than 100 mg a day or more to supposedly relatively mimic the benefits seen in laboratory animals. Be especially careful of sources. The *cis*-form of resveratrol is completely ineffective, but widely sold in commercial resveratrol supplements simply labeled "resveratrol." Read the label carefully

▸ CoQ10—helps support healthy mitochondrial function, serves as a powerful fat-soluble antioxidant, and can greatly improve oxygen and energy utilization. It is found in every major organ—especially the heart (and is dramatically and dangerously depleted by the use of statin drugs). (100–300 mg/day or more, if needed)

▸ Adequate intake of omega-3 fatty acids. Getting adequate amounts of this *critically important* vital nutrient often calms or eliminates carbohydrate cravings and greatly enhances insulin sensitivity

▸ L-glutamine, an amino acid, can stop cravings for sweets, starches and alcohol instantly, as the brain is able to use L-glutamine temporarily for fuel. It is also the #1 food for enterocytes, the cells lining the small intestine, and can greatly help regenerate gastro-intestinal mucosa. Usually comes in 500 mg capsules and needs to be taken on an empty stomach for best effect. Start with lowest dose and increase as necessary. Can also be absorbed sublingually (sprinkled under the tongue) for a more immediate effect. Up to two grams (2,000 mg) or even more may be necessary. Loose powders are widely available and quite palatable, if larger doses are needed. (Caution: refrain from using L-glutamine if you knowingly have cancer, as L-glutamine can serve to fuel certain types of tumor growth)

▸ The herb, *Gymnema sylvestre*, taken in 4-gram (4,000 mg) increments, three times a day can usually eliminate most, if not all, cravings for sweets. In extremely addicted individuals, twice this dose may be needed to successfully eliminate cravings. This is a great tool that can be likened to "bicycle training wheels" while dietary modifications are being made. After a time, this will no longer be needed once healthier eating habits are adopted. It also possesses compounds that may support the restoration of insulin sensitivity

▸ Eliminate the use of caffeine and other stimulants. Stimulants aggravate blood sugar problems and deplete important neurotransmitters, serotonin and norepinephrine, adversely affecting mood and energy

▸ Sometimes, a person craving carbohydrates is merely starved for adequate protein and, more specifically L-tryptophan, the least abundant amino acid in our food supply. Supplementing with appropriate doses of L-tryptophan can calm these cravings and help restore healthy neurotransmitter (serotonin) function. Start with one 500-mg capsule on an empty stomach and increase each half-hour until a feeling of increased well-being is achieved. DO NOT USE L-tryptophan if you are currently taking SSRIs or MAO inhibitors (antidepressants), except under guidance of a knowledgeable healthcare practitioner

▸ Try adding some pancreatic lipase on an empty stomach. Deficiencies of lipase are common in those who have trouble managing blood sugar and supplementation can improve your ability to digest and use fats instead of sugar for fuel! (Found typically as part of a pancreatic enzyme complex supplement)

▸ Seek to reduce or eliminate unnecessary use of over-the-counter and prescription medications

▸ Stop smoking. Duh!

▸ Eliminate the use of alcohol

▸ Avoid alternative "natural" sweeteners such as honey, rice syrup, lo han syrup, fructose, agave nectar and maple syrup.

▸ Stevia is a carbohydrate-free sweetener derived from a South

American herb. It is anywhere from 200–300 times sweeter than sugar and is therefore used only in very small amounts. Extracts containing "steviosides" (active herbal compounds) have been shown to benefit blood sugar stability. It is the only sugar substitute I am comfortable recommending for all but the most sugar-reactive individuals. Stevia is widely sold in health food stores and many supermarkets. It works very well in beverages and can be used in cooking. It can be purchased in refined form in packets, also in liquid extracts and as a powdered herb. The brand of Stevia I've found that is the least refined (short of growing it yourself in an herb garden, which many people do) is "Stevita" (www.stevitastevia.com). *Caution:* sweet tastes may foster sweet cravings

▸ Eliminate use of aspartame ("Nutrasweet"), sucrolose ("Splenda"), acesulfame-K ("Sweet-One"), saccharin ("Sweet-n-Low"), and all other artificial sweeteners. *Period.* Avoid them like the plague. Studies show these are more likely to make you fat than thin, as well as increasing your risk for cancer and numerous other health problems

▸ Eliminate all MSG. MSG, an excitotoxin, has been shown to directly cause leptin resistance and induce obesity, in addition to being markedly toxic to the brain

▸ Identify and eliminate foods to which you may be allergic or sensitive. This can be an extremely problematic source of cortisol-induced, unwanted insulin production and weight gain. Elimination/provocation diets are the gold standard and most affordable method of diagnosis. Grains (gluten) and dairy (casein) are the most common offenders, followed by soy, peanuts and corn. Chicken eggs are also commonly problematic for many A stool antibody test by Enterolab (www.enterolab.com) can be reliably diagnostic of several common food sensitivities, as well.

▸ Get a good night's sleep. Don't be a night owl. Studies repeatedly show sleep deprivation as strongly correlated with decreased insulin sensitivity and unwanted weight gain, along with other problems. Try to get at least 6–8 quality hours of sleep every single night, as we were designed to do!

► Do exercise daily, or at least 3–5 times per week. Short bouts of high intensity interval training and resistance training are most effective. Exercise has been shown to decidedly help improve insulin sensitivity. Exercise such as this immediately following a meal containing carbohydrates, also can help burn off some of the sugar

► Give special attention to stress management. Increased stress hormone levels (e.g. cortisol) also, sometimes greatly, enhance elevated blood sugar levels and insulin production, as well as suppress the immune system. *Actively cultivate stress reduction habits . . . or else!*

Note: Sugar, alcohol or carbohydrate cravings, as well as cravings for stimulants such as caffeine, are commonly a strong indication of serotonin depletion. Chronic use of these substances actually depletes serotonin over time and can lead to low levels of this important neurotransmitter. This may either generate or exacerbate cognitive deficits, as well as depressive, labile or anxious states—particularly in susceptible individuals (Schwarzbein, 1999).

Eleven more reasons to cut the carbs (if you aren't already convinced)

1. High-carbohydrate diets lower HDL cholesterol and, more importantly, raise triglycerides—an independent risk for heart attack
2. You are much more likely to suffer a heart attack following a high carbohydrate meal than a high fat meal
3. Carbohydrates raise insulin, which makes you fat and increases risk for, metabolic disorder, diabetes and worse
4. A high intake of carbohydrates and sweetened beverages is

associated with an increased risk of breast cancer (Witte et al, 1997)

5. Carbohydrates eaten in excess raise levels of plasminogen activator inhibitor-1, which increases risk of heart attacks and strokes

6. Eating too many carbohydrates makes LDL cholesterol smaller and denser, creating lipoprotein(a), which in turn raises risk of heart and artery disease. No statin drug can modify or reduce lipoprotein(a)—only diet (i.e., reduction of insulin provoking carbohydrates)

7. Eating a lot of starches and sugars raises levels of blood fats following a meal—a condition called postprandial lipemia—which is another risk factor for heart disease

8. Eating a lot of starches and sugars can increase the likelihood of yeast overgrowth, a toxic bowel, and impaired ability of the liver to remove toxic materials from the body, all of which increase risk of disease

9. Pregnant women who eat diets high in carbohydrates form smaller placentas (Godfrey et al, 1996). This has ominous implications. The formation of the placenta dictates how well the mother will be able to transfer nutrients to the fetus

10. A diet high in grains like wheat or legumes, which contain mostly starch, will contain phytates that reduce the absorption of valuable nutrients like calcium, iron and zinc. Such a diet will also increase your exposure to highly allergenic compounds such as gluten, found in wheat, rye, oats and barley, potentially even leading to autoimmune diseases

11. Excessive intake of carbohydrates, especially sugar, will weaken immune function. Too many carbohydrates also increase the damage that stress can do to the body (Holman, 1996).

(Adapted from *The Carnitine Miracle,* by Robert Crayhon, MA)

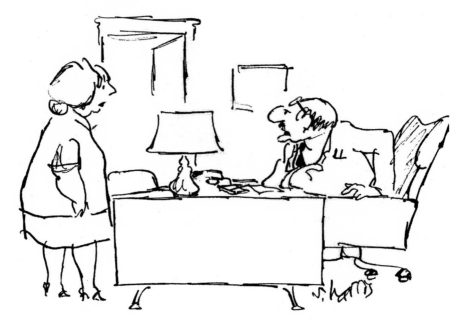

"LET ME PUT IT THIS WAY: YOU'RE AN ADDICT AND YOUR GROCER IS A PUSHER."

HIGH FRUCTOSE CORN SYRUP:
A STICKY WICKET BEST AVOIDED

Today, the number-one source of dietary calories in America comes from a corn-based industrial sweetener known as "high fructose corn syrup" (HFCS). It is an ingredient used to sweeten everything from sodas, cookies, soups, yogurt, salad dressing, bread, cereal, iced tea, "health bars," ketchup, bacon, peanut butter, mustard . . . even beer. It is prevalent in nearly *all* processed foods. Ninety cents out of every dollar in America spent on food is spent on processed food. The food industry uses HFCS more than any other sweetener because it's cheap to produce, transport and store.

It is among the most dangerous and damaging food additives ever created.

HFCS has been shown to interfere with a key enzyme in the body that delivers copper to your vital organs. This effectively results in copper deficiency for many, adversely impacting a wide range of organ systems including the heart, testes, pancreas, and damaging the liver—generating inflammation and cirrhosis. It has been strongly linked to the sharp rise in both obesity and diabetes. Furthermore, fructose is 20–30 times more glycating than glucose. It turns anyone into a raging AGE-producing factory. Animals fed a high-fructose diet in laboratory studies developed livers that looked a lot like those of hardcore, aging alcoholics—inflamed and shot through with dead cells and scar tissue—the condition known as "cirrhosis."

High fructose corn syrup has been linked to:
- Diabetes
- Heart disease
- Cancer
- Obesity
- Weakened immune system
- Cirrhosis of the liver
- Osteoporosis
- Elevated cholesterol
- Anemia
- Mineral deficiency

Read *all* labels . . . and avoid HFCS like the plague that it is. Beware of cheap, processed foods! The price you pay may be way higher than you think!

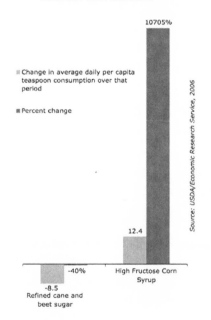

Change in use of High Fructose Corn Syrup between 1970 and 2005

"Be wary of all the chemicals in your life."
—ANDREW WEIL, MD

The Corn Refiners Association insists: "Research confirms that high fructose corn syrup is safe and no different from other common sweeteners like table sugar and honey. All three sweeteners are nutritionally the same." This, of course, is all part of the Corn Refiners Association's 20–30 million dollar advertising and public relations campaign to counter the overwhelming scientific evidence to the contrary. Reasearch findings since 2004 have been extremely damaging to the HFCS market, and justifiably so.

HFCS is metabolized into fat faster than almost any other sugar—augmented when in liquid form as found in soft drinks. Chemical tests among eleven different carbonated soft drinks containing HFCS were found to have "astonishingly high" levels of reactive carbonyls. Reactive carbonyls are undesirable and highly-reactive compounds associated with "unbound" fructose and glucose molecules, and are believed to cause tissue damage (via A.G.E.'s) that is known to also cause diabetes, according to new evidence found by recent research, reported at the 2007 national meeting of the American Chemical Society. Based on the study data, the researchers estimate that a single can of soda contains about five times the concentration of reactive carbonyls than the concentration found in the blood of an adult person with diabetes.

Additionally, all HFCS is manufactured from genetically modified (GMO) corn, which has been linked to a much higher incidence of corn related allergies, among other, more insidious problems potentially associated with any GMO food.

Finally, it has also recently been revealed that HFCS contains significant traces of mercury—an extremely powerful and damaging neurotoxin (and, yes—the FDA knew and did nothing).

Read all labels. Avoid HFCS like the plague that it is, and beware of cheap, processed foods. The price you pay may be much higher than you think!

What about artificial sweeteners?

Chemical substitutes for sugar such as Aspartame (Nutrasweet), Sucralose (Splenda), Acesulfame-K (Sunnette), and Saccharine (Sweet-n-Low) have all been implicated in innumerable, serious problems and symptoms and should not be used by anyone who cares about their health. More consumer complaints have been filed against Nutrasweet, alone, than any other substance governed by the FDA, and a recent study conducted from the Duke University Medical Center published in September of 2008 in the *Journal of Toxicology and Environmental Health* (Drs. Mohamed B. Abou-Donia, Eman M. El-Masry, Ali A. Abdel-Rahman, Roger E. McLendon and Susan S. Schiffman) indicates that Splenda® reduces the amount of good bacteria in the intestines by 50%, increases the pH level in the intestines, contributes to increases in body weight and affects the P-glycoprotein (P-gp) in the body in such a way that crucial cancer/HIV-related drugs could be rejected and critical nutrients in general may not be absorbed. This is only one recent study among many illustrating considerable reason for concern and avoidance of these sugar substitutes.

All artificial sweeteners have been implicated in cancer (among many other things), and none are naturally occurring substances in nature. They should all be avoided by everyone. The only sugar substitute that seems to be entirely safe is the South American herb, Stevia. Stevia is about 300 times sweeter than sugar, has no carbohydrate or caloric value, has been safely used by primitive South American cultures for centuries and may even have some beneficial glucose regulating and insulin sensitivity-restoring effects.

> **Remember: if it comes out of a test tube it's not food.**

WHY YOU SHOULDN'T USE THE "GLYCEMIC INDEX" AS YOUR GUIDE

The glycemic index was established as a means of gauging how rapidly the sugar in various foods enters the bloodstream as compared to pure glucose (or white bread). Glucose, or white bread, is assigned an arbitrary value of 100, against which all other foods are measured. Other foods are assigned a number that reflects a percentage of that glucose rating. The higher the percentage, the bigger the surge in blood sugar the food causes, the more it raises insulin and the more potentially problematic it may be.

Seems like a useful thing, right?

Well . . . the problems with this method of measuring the effect of sugar in food are many. First, there are actually two different ways in which a food can be "low glycemic." First, it can be like fiber, which simply doesn't have any sugar content or convert to sugar in the body. Or it can be like fructose, which doesn't have much impact on insulin, but it is an extremely glycating—or, more properly in this instance, "fructosilating"—substance that can do immeasurable damage to your arteries and tissues. In fact, fructose is twenty to thirty times *more glycating* than glucose.

Interestingly, some foods actually have a higher glycemic index score than glucose. Puffed rice, corn flakes, Rice Krispies and instant white rice all rank higher (Run, don't walk away from these foods . . . and don't look back.).

The glycemic index is always based upon 50 grams of a particular carbohydrate. So, although, say, a carrot may have a rather high glycemic index, this does not take into account the fiber, water, vitamins or minerals in that carrot. It actually boils down to being a fairly modest amount of actual sugar per carrot; this varies further depending on whether the carrots are cooked or not. Cooked carrots are significantly more glycemic than raw . . . another thing the glycemic index may not take into account. If you wanted to get the effect from carrots that are reflected by the glycemic index, you'd need to eat twelve to thirteen carrots in a sitting. That's a lot of carrots—though something more easily exceeded if you happen to be juicing those carrots.

Another thing the index does not take into account is what other foods you are eating with that particular food; that may greatly alter its glycemic effect. Finally, the glycemic index is based upon a limited window of only three hours and does not take into effect certain foods, such as, say, alcohol sugars, that have a delayed glycemic effect and impact blood sugar much later—something not understood until recently.

The glycemic index doesn't really tell you how much "utilizable carbohydrate" exists in a particular food, which leads to being a very misleading gauge. Using another method of gauging carbohydrate content of a food like *glycemic load*—is a bit more useful—still takes the glycemic index into account but is based instead on a per-serving standard, which is far more realistic and practical. Glycemic load is calculated by taking the assigned glycemic index number, dividing it by 100, and then multiplying it by the actual grams of carbs in a particular serving size.

This is a slightly better approach, though it's far from perfect. It still won't take into account the impact of fructose or alcohol sugars, cooking methods or other foods that may be combined with the food in question. For that, you are on your own and must simply use your own awareness and best judgment. Avoiding utilizable carbohydrate as much as possible should be the default rule. This isn't to say you shouldn't be eating carrots, but it's better not to overdo them. The lower the sugar and/or starch content of your veggies, the better!

WHAT ABOUT FIBER AS AN "ESSENTIAL" CARBOHYDRATE?

ABC World News Tonight with Peter Jennings reported on January 20, 1999: "Massive study reports fiber 'worthless' in helping to prevent colon cancer." The study had just been released in the *New England Journal of Medicine.* The report found that fiber, once thought to be a panacea for preventing colon cancer, provides no protection at all from the disease. The study, described as a massive nurses' study involving 88,000 people, and spanning sixteen years, stated conclusively that consuming a high-fiber diet makes no difference whatsoever in prevention of colon cancer.

Cultures such as the Inuit, as well as Ice Age humans, consumed little or no dietary fiber. This isn't to say that certain antioxidants and nutrients found in vegetables and fruits aren't of value to us or that fiber has no useful role at all to play. Clearly, great varieties of fibrous vegetables and fruits have been typically abundant in healthy primitive hunter-gatherer societies, following the last Ice Age through today, and their antioxidants are probably more important to us now than ever. Fiber does not appear to be a critical part of the equation, however, and vegetables and fruits are not the be-all and end-all.

It is clear from other anthropological evidence and other studies that fiber, from vegetables and fruits, may not be as central to our health and longevity as nutritional—particularly vegetarian or vegan—pundits would have us believe. In fact, excess dietary fiber can serve to excessively bind minerals in the diet, irritate the colon (particularly fiber from grains) and create significant mineral deficiencies.

On the plus-side, *soluble* fiber (found in nuts, seeds, fibrous vegetables and fruit) may serve to feed healthy bacteria in the gut (assuming, of course, one has healthy bacteria in the gut to feed) which they may then convert to useful nutrients substances such as butyric acid—the primary fuel for colon cells and the #1 colon cancer-preventing substance, along with vitamins A and D. Incidentally, butyric acid is also richly found in grass-fed butter, and is partly where butyric acid actually gets its name. Butter—also a superb source of true vitamin A—may in fact be a greater preventative food for colon cancer than dietary fiber ever could be. Who knew?

The sun and vitamin D, however, may be the best colon cancer preventative of all. Dr. Gordon Ainsleigh, a sunlight advocate, encourages sunbathing to foster healthy vitamin D levels to fight cancer. In 1992, Ainsleigh reviewed fifty years' worth of medical literature on cancer and the sun. He reported in the journal *Preventive Medicine* that widespread, regular, moderate sunbathing would lower the incidence of breast and colon cancer death rates by a whopping one-third.

Fiber can be useful in helping bind spent, conjugated hormones in the gut and eliminating them before they can be re-absorbed. In a world where we are living in a sea of dangerously excessive estrogen and estrogen-like compounds termed "xenoestrogens," fiber has probably never been more useful in this regard than it is now.

When it comes right down to it, though, probably the best thing about fiber is that it doesn't convert to sugar.

So go ahead and eat your veggies—and plenty of them—with melted butter or olive oil, to help better absorb the minerals and fat-soluble nutrients in them. Lightly sautéing or steaming can also help break down cellulose, improving digestibility. Limit fruits, due to their sugar content (some antioxidant-rich berries are okay). Fibrous vegetables are nicely filling and we need the extra antioxidants and phytonutrients they may provide us, especially in today's toxic world. Just remember, fibrous vegetables may just be a side dish—but they are an important one in modern times—in fact, probably more now than ever.

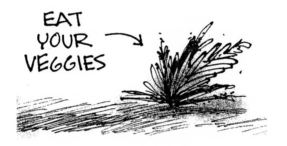

WHAT ABOUT JUICING—
ISN'T THAT REALLY GOOD FOR YOU?

The whole idea around juicing seems healthy enough: get more servings per day of fruits and vegetables into yourself by juicing them and getting rid of the indigestible pulp. It's all the rage in health food stores and health clubs, and a fad that borders on prescriptive dogma among devout health nuts and vegans. Nice plan, on the surface of things, but what are you actually doing? *Think!*

For starters, our ancestors never would have done such a thing. They always ate the *whole* vegetable or piece of fruit, discarding mainly any woody stems or seeds. The idea of extracting and discarding the pulp and drinking the liquid from vegetables or fruits is quite unnatural and makes a very flawed assumption: that the bulk of the nutritional content of these foods exists in the juice.

Unfortunately, that's just wrong.

Consider, for instance, that the skin of any fruit or vegetable is what actually protects the vital interior components from the ravages of the environment, including radiation. As such, *the greater concentration of antioxidants in any fruit or vegetable is almost always in the skin.* The pulp also contains numerous bioflavinoids, pigments and phytonutrients, which also get discarded typically in juicing. So, what are you left with in the liquid? *Mostly sugar water* mixed with a few vitamins, minerals and diluted amounts of other nutrients. Tasty, but the negative impact of the sugar will outweigh whatever benefits are received from the other nutrients in the juice almost every time.

It's not that some of what lies in the juice isn't good for you . . . it's just that the sugar is always worse.

Juicing low-glycemic, fibrous vegetables and greens, on the other hand, is perfectly okay—even quite beneficial—as their sugar content is minimal. Steer away from sweetening it with too much carrot juice, though. It's better just to eat those whole and raw. Add something like Stevia, if you have to.

If you want to juice your fruits, that's great. Just throw out the sugar water and eat the pulp instead!

ADRENAL EXHAUSTION:
A UNIQUELY MODERN EPIDEMIC

Among the most common modern-day afflictions—both diagnosed by holistic practitioners and undiagnosed—is what is known as "adrenal exhaustion." This is brought about by chronic or severe stress, chronic exposure to food sensitivities; electromagnetic frequency (EMFs); pollution from cell phones, cordless phones, wi-fi, and other electro-pollution; and especially excess dietary carbohydrate and blood sugar dysregulation. Adrenal stress, dysregulation and/or exhaustion can leave you feeling completely worn out, depleted and can greatly interfere with normal sleep patterns. The symptoms of low adrenal function are varied, depending on severity and individual factors, and can commonly include:

- Trouble staying asleep
- Being a "slow starter" in the morning
- Afternoon fatigue
- Feeling run down or overwhelmed
- Salt and sweet cravings
- Experiencing dizziness when standing up too quickly
- Afternoon headaches or headaches with stress or exertion

Adrenal dysregulation can also include adrenal "hyperfunction" (not to be confused with Cushing's disease), which may eventually also lead to some stage of adrenal exhaustion. Common symptoms of adrenal hyperfunction can include:

- ► Feeling constantly "stressed out"
- ► Trouble falling asleep
- ► Irritability and anxiety
- ► High blood sugar
- ► Tending toward weight gain under stress
- ► Excess perspiration, or perspiring even while inactive (in normal temperatures)
- ► Waking up tired, seemingly no matter what

Adrenaline is the hormone secreted by the adrenal medulla associated with acute states of "flight or fight." Once released, it mobilizes blood sugar to fuel the "emergency," dilates pupils, shuts down digestion and other "non-essential" or "non-survival"-oriented bodily functions, constricts blood vessels, raising blood pressure, and increases the heart rate. Cortisol, secreted by the adrenal cortex, is produced in response to more chronic states of stress and as a blood sugar management hormone. Individuals with chronic stress and/or dysglycemia may exhaust the adrenal cortex's ability to produce adequate cortisol (see ASI example #1) and result in what can be termed "adrenal exhaustion."

As leptin rules the endocrine roost, as it were, and insulin stands firmly second in command, the adrenal hormones, adrenaline and cortisol, are next in the line of authority over your moods, energy and well-being. The health of your thyroid depends on the health of your adrenals. In fact, no thyroid issue can ever fully resolve without the restoration of adrenal health.

Women must depend upon healthy adrenals to ease the transition of menopause. Exhausted adrenals are unable to take the "baton" from the ovaries, as they are supposed to at this time, to continue producing needed hormones. If your adrenals are shot, that "transition" called menopause can be pure hell. Women with healthy adrenals at menopause barely even notice anything has happened . . . which is how it is supposed to be.

Your adrenals are often the first obvious casualty of blood sugar dysregulation. Stymied adrenal function can lead to chronic feelings of stress, fatigue, being overwhelmed, weight gain, insomnia, mood disorders or instability, headaches or migraines and eventually thyroid problems. (Down the road, sex hormone problems can develop, too, via an endocrine metabolic phenomenon known as the "pregnenelone steal"). *You will never correct a problem with your thyroid or sex hormones without first correcting adrenal imbalance.* And in order to correct that, of course, you must determine and address your main adrenal stressors and address issues around insulin and leptin.

Common adrenal stressors can include blood sugar dysregulation (the big one), the chronic use of stimulants, chronic high levels of EMF exposure, food sensitivity issues, prolonged life stress or chronic trauma, chronic lack of adequate sleep and/or excessive exercise.

Apart from excess dietary carbohydrates and lifestyle issues, the second most common cause of adrenal problems is easily food sensitivities. (See chapter: "What about Food Allergies and Sensitivities?") Consuming food substances to which you are sensitive will automatically generate a stress response in the body that involves both cortisol and insulin. Even if your diet is low carb and/or low cal, it is possible to gain undesirable weight and generate systemic inflammation, chronically eating foods to which one is intolerant.

There are several vicious cycles that may be commonly generated from adrenal dysregulation that can be difficult to correct. The hypothalamic-pituitary-adrenal axis can become dysregulated, leading to many other hormonal problems. The hippocampus of the brain—needed for emotional/neurological stability, short term memory and memory consolidation, among other things—can begin degenerating due to excess cortisol saturation and excess "excitatory activity" that can include chronic stress, EMF pollution (a topic covered later), not getting enough sleep, excess dietary carbohydrates and food sensitivities. Also, the GI tract may suffer impaired regenerative capacity and/or mucosal erosion due to either insufficient or excess cortisol levels, which can lead to "leaky gut," allergies, immune vulnerabilities and food sensitivities . . . among other things. The popular use of progesterone creams can also create or exacerbate cortisol excesses.

Excess leptin and insulin surges generated by chronic carbohydrate consumption can get this problematic adrenal ball rolling in no small way and create a self-perpetuating nightmare.

Suffice it to say, it ain't pretty. These vicious cycles can unravel anyone.

Cortisol levels shift throughout the day naturally and follow a predictable daily rhythmic pattern that can become dysregulated by stress. These "pattern disruptions" (see ASI example #2) may be readily managed by the use of "adaptogens," which are typically certain herbs that can help re-set these erratic patterns on a "brain communication" level and restore healthy cortisol rhythms. An Adrenal Stress Index, or ASI, is a salivary hormone panel (via the lab Diagnos-Techs, Inc.) offered by many Certified Nutritional Therapists, Nutritional Therapy Practitioners, Naturopaths and other holistic practitioners, and can be used to accurately evaluate adrenal function and cortisol rhythms. (*Note:* efforts to support adrenal recovery may be entirely futile with individuals who are anemic. The presence of anemia must first be ruled out and/or properly addressed when seeking to support adrenal issues).

Examples of ASI Results:

Example #1

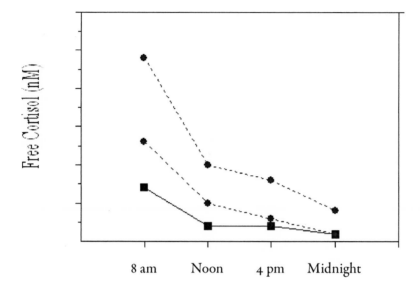

Example #1 above: a dysregulated cortisol pattern, as revealed by an ASI.

The dark, black line connected by squares shows the person's actual pattern (in this case, depressed cortisol levels and "stage 7" adrenal exhaustion), while dotted lines reflect the upper and lower limits of normal, healthy cortisol range at various points during the day, early morning through nighttime. This person experiences chronic fatigue and regularly craves caffeine.

Example #2

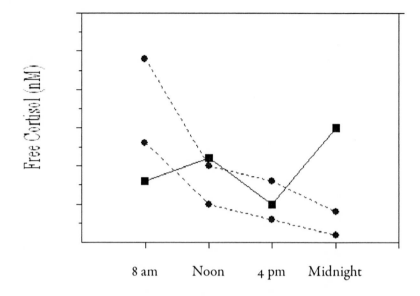

Example #2: a dysregulated cortisol pattern.

The pattern in example #2 reflects a markedly dysregulated corti-sol rhythm throughout the day and night and may respond well to supplementation with adaptogens. This person experiences extreme fatigue in the morning (craving caffeine) and problems with restless sleep and winding down at night.

Once properly evaluated, steps may be taken to appropriately sup-port the specific adrenal issues and help bring them back into balance. Beware of recommendations that include hormonal replacement, however. Hormones such as DHEA and/or pregnenolone should *only* be considered in cases of what is known as "stage 7" adrenal exhaus-tion, only taken in very minute amounts as a liquid sublingual prepa-ration and only for short periods of time.

Otherwise, please resist direct hormonal "supplementation"— even "bio-identical"—unless there is absolutely no other choice. This should only be considered a last resort. Remember: *Hormones are* not *supplements.*

Addressing the body functionally, as a whole, taking into account the extreme complexity of its biochemical or hormonal inter-relationships, is the most effective way to actually correct the underlying problem and achieve long-term restoration of health. Dealing with each component of health, endocrine or body function as a separate entity only leads to more imbalances in the long run—and big bank accounts for the practitioners who subscribe to this archaic and outmoded approach. Functional medicine and nutritional therapy—that takes into account the intricate complexity of human systems and evaluates from a foundational standpoint—is the clear and necessary future of positive health management.

When addressing adrenal issues, always first consider the endocrine chain of command and be aware that in order to correct imbalances you must always look first "upstream" and consider what may have caused the initial imbalance in the first place. Modern conventional medicine, often even holistic medicine, is quick to micro-manage hormonal issues they are willing to recognize by prescribing hormone replacement. (Note that MDs tend not to recognize "adrenal imbalances" that are not full-blown diseases.) Even "bio-identical" hormone replacement can be extremely problematic when utilized in this way. This is not to say that bio-identical hormone replacement is never necessary, but it also shouldn't necessarily always be the first step in resolving imbalances. Inter-relationships with other hormones must also be carefully considered.

Look to the source. Go to the foundations first—always.

A WORD ABOUT WATER

Chronic cellular dehydration painfully and prematurely kills. Its initial outward manifestations have until now been labeled as diseases of unknown origin.
—F. BATMANGHELIDJ, MD, 1995

Water is literally the most important substance we put into our bodies, next to oxygen. Most of us fail to get enough of it. It is utilized in literally *every* metabolic process in the human body and is utterly essential to the function of the human brain and nervous system. The human body mass is comprised of roughly 55–60% water and the human brain up to 70–80%. The human body can produce about 8% of its water needs from its own metabolic processes. That leaves a remaining 92% that must be obtained through diet. Caffeinated beverages and alcohol cause dehydration, as does stress and physical activity. Replenishing the body with substantial amounts of pure, clean water is critical. No nutrient in the body can function without water. And the body's bioelectrical system is non-existent without it. Often, what may seem like complex physical or emotional issues may be little more than chronic dehydration. As little as a 2% loss of our body's water content through diuresis or dehydration can result in noticeable fatigue. A drop of 10% can cause problems ranging from musculoskeletal issues (e.g., joint pain, back pain, cramps), to digestive problems (e.g., heartburn, constipation), immune problems or allergies, and even cardiovascular symptoms or anginal pain.

The importance of this foundational substance, essential to all life should never, ever be underestimated.

Save your money by avoiding sodas, juices and other either unnatural or unnecessary, or sugary, beverages. Water is always best. And it's affordable. Dehydrating beverages include caffeine, alcohol, some herbal teas, all juices and sodas. Be sure to add another 12–16 ounces of pure water to your daily intake, for every 8 ounces of diuretic beverage consumed. For further excellent information, look for the book: *Your Body's Many Cries for Water*, by F. Batmanghelidj, MD. Also see the Web site: www.watercure.com. Stay away from plastic bottles as much as possible and stick to non-chemical-leeching reusable or refillable containers to store your portable water supply.

Symptoms potentially associated with chronic dehydration:

- Depression
- Stress
- Dyspeptic pain
- Colitis pain
- False appendicitis pain
- Hiatus hernia
- Rheumatoid arthritis pain
- Low back pain
- Neck pain
- Anginal pain
- Anxiety
- Headaches
- High blood pressure
- High blood cholesterol
- Excess body weight
- Excess hunger
- Asthma and allergies
- Chronic fatigue
- Irritability
- Constipation
- Cognitive impairment

Feeling symptomatic? If in doubt, try drinking a tall glass of pure, clean, filtered water!

UNDERSTANDING THE ROLE OF PROTEIN

Protein is essential to life and, unlike carbohydrates, is essential to diet. Although we are able to synthesize and recycle many proteins and amino acids—our body is made up of over 50,000+ different proteins—there are eight amino acids, the building blocks of protein, known to be "essential": leucine, isoleucine, valine, lysine, phenylalanine, tryptophan, threonine and methionine. "Essential" basically means these cannot be made in the body and *must* be derived from dietary sources and fully present for normal protein synthesis to occur in the body. Without the presence of *complete* protein in the diet, normal healthy protein synthesis in our body is brought to a screeching halt.

Quality complete protein is exclusively found in animal source foods.

Combining vegetarian protein sources in order to create complete protein, such as beans and brown rice, for instance, still makes for a dominantly starchy food, yielding far more sugar than protein; despite the combined more "complete" amino acid profile, in no way does this imply protein *sufficiency*. To accomplish actual daily protein sufficiency with rice and beans, the trade-off would be excessive caloric intake to meet the protein demand from a more carbohydrate or starch-based food source. The result yields disastrous implications for blood sugar regulation, together with excess insulin and leptin surges.

Hot off the press

In just the last couple of years, a brand new and extremely important metabolic pathway was discovered no one previously knew was there. Researchers were studying a naturally occurring substance known as *rapimycin* (synthesized from soil bacteria), as it was able to demonstrate some fairly powerful cancer-inhibiting properties. Drug companies were extremely interested in finding out how it worked and accidentally stumbled across this new, previously unknown metabolic pathway, now referred to as *mTOR,* which stands for "mammalian target of rapimycin."

Much as insulin serves as a sort of default "sugar sensor" and leptin serves as our body's "fat sensor," mTOR (it turns out) *serves as our body's protein sensor,* monitoring the availability of protein, or amino acids (particularly the branched chain amino acids), for growth and reproduction. It is also influenced by insulin levels and is part of a related metabolic pathway. When protein levels are detected that exceed our basic maintenance requirements, this up-regulates the mTOR pathway, stimulating cellular proliferation. Increased insulin also has this effect and the mTOR protein belongs to what is known as the P13K pathway that is activated by insulin, nutrients and growth factors. mTOR has a central role in the regulation of cell growth and protein synthesis. It essentially activates our reproductive capacity.

Again, cellular proliferation occurs mainly under three circumstances: reproduction (DNA replication), growth, as, for example, in children, . . . and cancer. A presentation on April 14, 2008, at the American Association for Cancer Research annual meeting revealed that modified caloric restriction may offer a protective effect against the development of epithelial cancers. Epithelial cancers, also known as carcinomas, arise in the tissue that lines the surfaces and cavities of the body's organs, and make up 80% of all cancers. "Calorie restriction and obesity directly affect activation of the cell surface receptors epidermal growth factor and insulin-like growth factor," explained study coauthor Tricia Moore, a graduate student in MD Anderson's Department of Carcinogenesis. "These receptors then affect signaling in downstream molecular pathways such as Akt and mTOR. Calorie restriction, which we refer to as negative energy balance, inhibits this signaling, and obesity, or positive energy balance, enhances signaling through these pathways, leading to cell growth, proliferation and survival."

If, however, the dietary protein level stays below this threshold, ancient mechanisms kick in that are designed to help us outlive an "apparent famine," which then shuts down cellular proliferation and up-regulates, instead, repair and regeneration. It signals an effort to keep us healthy enough, long enough so that our cells may reproduce another day. That's what we want. We want just enough protein to meet the demands of our own repair, regeneration and basic maintenance needs that can extend our own longevity, enhance our own health and possibly even reverse signs of aging . . . but not so much that we up-regulate mTOR. And we always want to keep insulin levels as low as possible.

So . . . how much is "just enough"? For most adults the RDA, 46–53 grams of protein per day is probably sufficient (one of the rare RDAs worth following). An extremely athletic, large person under tremendous physical demand or someone particularly depleted nutritionally may possibly need up to 60 or 70 grams. . . . Just maybe. This amounts to just a few ounces of concentrated, complete protein per day (see protein content in foods chart at the back of this book), best consumed in divided amounts. Just as an example, a single tin of sardines in olive oil yields about 27 grams of protein (plus lots of high-quality fats, including EPA/DHA) . . . just about half your total daily needs! That's about all. It's not a lot, and it's far fewer grams of protein than many people regularly consume—even per meal.

The key here is *nutrient density per calorie.* Quality and digestibility of the protein source is key and matters more than quantity. This healthy modification to your diet alone can readily save you thousands on grocery bills, while still allowing you to afford the best quality, nutrient dense sources (e.g., fully grass-fed, organic and/or wild caught) of protein.

Keeping protein consumption to a much more moderate level also makes digesting it far less challenging. You are more apt to easily digest and make better use of a small amount of protein at a meal, as opposed to a large slab of meat or fish in your gut that your body has to struggle with breaking down and assimilating. Many lack sufficient hydrochloric acid and pancreatic enzymes to do so; lesser amounts of protein ease the digestive burden. Protein digestion is also very energy intensive—in fact, digestion demands more energy than anything else we do—and moderating intake may improve energy levels and help

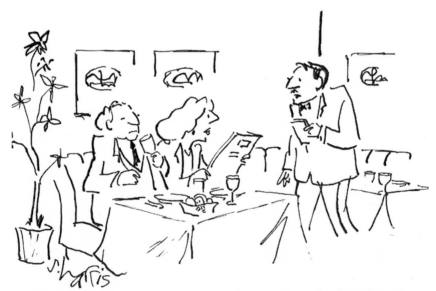

"WOULD YOU LIKE THAT TO BE A STEAK WITH A BROAD-SPECTRUM ANTIBIOTIC, OR ONE WITH A VARIETY OF THERAPEUTIC PROTEINS?"

minimize fatigue. Furthermore, the digestion of protein yields nitrogen by-products that the liver must process, which also burdens the eliminative system somewhat. Minimizing this also helps your body's eliminative processes function more efficiently, allowing for better detoxification, overall.

But isn't eating lots of lean protein what our ancestors did?

Protein—and food, in general—was not always as abundant as it is in our modern world. In more primitive times, we expended a fair amount of energy procuring it and there were times we had to live without adequate food for days, weeks and even months. Fat, as a key nutrient-rich energy source, was greatly coveted. Protein, too, was treated by our bodies as a precious commodity and was and is allocated carefully within our metabolic framework. Adequate dietary fat, by the way, is needed in order for protein to be properly utilized in the body. Nothing by our bodies is ever wasted. We have the ability to recycle a significant amount of protein in our bodies day to day, but we still need a few ounces of complete (i.e., animal-source) protein in our daily dietary intake.

If dietary protein is overly abundant, then dietary excesses are readily converted to sugar and stored as fat as a means of surviving what could be a future famine—and our metabolic pathways governing growth and reproduction are up-regulated, allowing for having children or storing fat. At the same time, these reproductive pathways are up-regulated; our own internal repair and maintenance pathways are down-regulated. "Out with the old, and in with the new," as it were.

When food is overly abundant and we eat that way, our ancient reproductive mechanisms recognize a window of opportunity for reproduction and basically somewhat sacrifice existing cellular repair and our own individual longevity interests for the sake of creating something new . . . and cellular proliferation ensues. But when food appears to the body as scarce, it's like saying, "Building a new house is too expensive right now . . . let's fix up the one we've got." The body up-regulates repair and regeneration, so we can stay healthy enough long enough to reproduce another day. It's a means of basically beating Mother Nature at her own game (something modern research can help us with that our Stone Age ancestors didn't know about). There are but two nutrients that directly mitigate this primordially-based biochemical decision-making process: carbohydrates (sugar) and protein. The pathways that regulate them are insulin and mTOR.

Why, you ask, is that?

OUR PRIMORDIAL PAST

Sugar and protein have been regulating reproduction and lifespan ever since the first single-celled organisms appeared in the earliest primordial seas. Glucose was life's first fuel on earth. This is all still a part of our genetic makeup, and the makeup of every other living organism on earth. It is an important fact to remember.

In this ancient time, when life in the form of single-celled organisms first appeared in the primordial seas—before there ever was an oxygen-based atmosphere—there were only two nutrients available: sugar and protein. These two nutrients established the basis of reproduction for all organisms, and, consequently, aging and lifespan. All energy production then was fermentative and anaerobic.

The first living cells were prokaryotic in nature—each one was identical to the next, like bacteria, for instance, lacked a nucleus and fed anaerobically on sugars.

Later, development of an oxygen-based atmosphere allowed for the evolution into eukaryotic cells (possessing a nucleus), which made cellular differentiation into organs, eyes, skin, etc. and higher organisms possible. The presence of oxygen allowed for the use of fat as a nutrient for the first time. Eukaryotic cells are fueled aerobically and utilize fatty acids for this purpose, just as most human and other mammalian cells do today. Fat is an "aerobic nutrient."

One theory of how cancers develop involves the idea that an excessively fermentative, acidic, sugar-rich and anaerobic environment somehow simulates our earliest primordial environment and stimulates the reversion of some cells to their primordial, prokaryotic state. Tumors are basically masses of undifferentiated identical cells with a weak protein matrix that feed exclusively on sugars. In other words, when the environment is ripe—when the availability of sugar is high and a fermentative, acidic, anaerobic environment is allowed to take hold—this primordial component of our genetic makeup is somehow triggered and stimulates cells into an unhealthy and exceedingly primitive form of cellular proliferation. Healthy cellular differentiation cannot occur in a fermentative environment. This certainly presents a plausible model for carcinogenesis, as well as other unhealthy forms of cellular proliferation.

The development of an oxygen-based atmosphere importantly allowed for the utilization of fat as an energy source. In the evolution of more complex organisms such as mammals, it is fat that serves as the primary, efficient source of fuel. Leptin, then—the key "fat sensor" in the body—controls and regulates all our energy stores via the hypothalamus, which manages the signals given to every other hormone in the body.

No matter what, leptin is always key.

UNDERSTANDING MOTHER NATURE'S PLAN AND WHERE WE FIT IN

As fundamentally primal beings, we have a well-developed survival instinct. We have an innate, vested interest in our own personal longevity and well-being. But we also harbor within us another influential entity with its own selfish agenda: our genes. Our genes are guided by nature's ultimate agenda (the big "A"), which is the perpetuation and continuity of Life (the big "L") as a Whole. This imperative also drives us to reproduce, as is the sole focus of those genes, whose sole purpose is simply to replicate.

Nature, it turns out, is not necessarily so interested in the things that constitute the individual components of life, such as you or me. We, as individual life forms, are but infinitesimal and ultimately expendable specks of dust in Mother Nature's bigger equation. Just as we have a basic indifference to the various cells in our own bodies that regularly degenerate and die, making way for new ones—all we care about, after all, is our overall survival and continuation—nature is primarily interested in its own ongoing big picture. Not, specifically, ours. Basically nature wants us to live long enough, and be healthy enough, so that we can reproduce successfully. Once we have achieved this end, or have arrived at the end of our useful reproductive life . . . well, it's not that nature wants us dead, necessarily . . . Nature sort of just loses interest.

Nature isn't that interested in innately guiding each of us how to live into very old age with health and vitality. That's where our own personal survival instinct—and modern science—come into play. We can't really count on nature's example to guide us here, or even the example of Stone Age humans, entirely. Eating foods that closely replicate the same diet that essentially shaped our physiological requirements, of course, makes inherent sense and must certainly play an essential role. But nature does not necessarily guide us to manipulate these dietary nutrients innately with post-reproductive longevity in mind. With respect to enhancing our post-reproductive longevity, we're basically on our own—without a fully natural compass.

What we are really seeking as individuals with our own personal drive toward survival, then, is to somehow find and exploit Mother Nature's loopholes for the benefit of our own individual post-reproductive health, longevity and expanded youth. For literally the first exciting time in our human history, we have the science available to tell us how to do exactly that.

Back in the 1930s, '40s and '50s, a number of experiments involving caloric restriction in animal models showed us that caloric restriction had a mysteriously universal effect of greatly improving health and extending lifespan. This research now spans some seventy-five years and is extremely well established and widely known.

Evidence of the effects of caloric restriction to slow aging and extend youth can be found in its abilities to prevent the immune dysfunctions of old age, improve DNA repair, reduce damaging free-radical activity, lower glucose and insulin levels, maintain fertility at advanced ages, boost energy levels, increase protein synthesis, reduce the accumulation of damaged proteins, inhibit the inflammatory responses of aging, lower blood levels of cholesterol and triglycerides, counteract neuro-degeneration and prevent the age-related decline in the health-building hormone dehydroepiandrosterone (DHEA).

Caloric restriction also prevents, postpones the incidence of, and reduces the severity of diseases such as cancer, kidney disease and cardiovascular disease (Masoro, EJ, 2003).

It is also known today to be additionally important that adequate vitamins, minerals and nutrients be added to caloric restriction approaches to avoid nutrient deficiencies. **The idea is to limit calories, not nutrients** (Nicolas, et al, 1999). Therefore, too, nutrient density plays an important role.

Longevity enthusiasts who attempt to apply this original research by attempting to sustain themselves each day on a single kumquat and a tablespoon of oatmeal are gravely missing the point, to say nothing of suffering an unnecessarily deprivation-oriented quality of life. No such thing is necessary . . . nor is it really helping them meet their hopeful objective. Recently popularized raw food vegan diets can achieve temporary improvements, by essentially down-regulating insulin and mTOR. The problem here is multi-fold, however.-In addition to the fact that we as humans lack four-stomachs and cud-chewing tendencies to maximize use of plant-based foods to meet all our needs, such a diet completely fails to provide many essential animal source nutrients needed for long-term maintenance of health, the brain/nervous system and vitality. Without adequate fat to normalize leptin (among countless other things) or complete protein sources to allow for critical re-building and maintenance such dietary approaches ultimately do far more harm than good, in the long run. The addition of quality raw animal food sources to these regimens would exponentially improve their long-term effectiveness.

To depict the more modern-day caloric restriction concept in science more accurately, the acronym, CRON—caloric restriction with optimal nutrition—has been suggested. "Under-nutrition without malnutrition" has been shown to consistently lengthen life span and postpone the onset of aging, cancer and degenerative diseases. Only carbohydrates and protein need to be limited (in that order), while fat and fat soluble nutrients actually play a more nutritionally and energetically dominant and supportive role.

The addition of antioxidant nutrients has been shown to have a potentially longevity enhancing effect on caloric restriction—something to additionally consider (Lemon, et al, 2005). Anti-glycating nutrients (benfotiamine, pyridoxamine, R-Lipoic acid, acetyl L-carnitine, L-carnosine, etc.) may also be considered additionally helpful for some.

Early on, it was believed (due to some flawed experiments involving macronutrient isolation) that it was caloric restriction, *in general* and not due to any one specific form of nutrient restriction that was somehow responsible for the effect. Feeding experiments in which lab rats were fed a diet exclusively consisting of carbohydrates led to rapid degeneration, accelerated aging, and death. Exclusive protein feeding also resulted in fairly rapid, degenerative decline and death.

Then researchers fed these rats a diet exclusively consisting of pure lard, an unnatural food for rats. Something different happened. Instead of developing degenerative diseases and cancer like the others, these rats developed impacted colons and their intestines ruptured. That—not any natural cause—is what killed them. Since the scientific community, as a whole, was on an active, rabid campaign of fat vilification during this time period, the fact that these rats died only confirmed what was essentially "expected" by the researchers, who just "knew" that fat was evil, anyway, and the actual *cause* of death was disregarded as insignificant.

This, of course, is outright lousy and fundamentally flawed science. The data concerning fat should either have been disregarded, or some new experiment devised. The flaws in this original research involving macronutrient manipulation have since been recognized, and we now know that fat factors differently into the equation. Until very recently, however, the mechanisms behind caloric restriction and why it actually worked were poorly understood.

Modern studies of healthy human centenarians, those 100 years old and older, have revealed the presence of a certain gene that seemed to be activated in these individuals. Called "sirtuins," they have come to be known as our "longevity gene." In mammals, this gene is referred to as *SIRT-1* (in worms it is called *SIR-2*). In certain fortunate people who appear to age unusually gracefully and remain vital to extremely old age, these SIRT-1 genes just sort of seem to be inherently activated, for unknown lucky reasons. This is why certain long-lived persons can claim to have not taken particular care of their health and still seem to make it to very old age. Such mysteriously fortunate individuals, of course, are the exception and not the rule. Recently, a nutrient found in red wine called resveratrol was shown to have the effect of stimulating this gene. It has also been clearly demonstrated that caloric restriction similarly activates these genes in all organisms and has all the same beneficial effects.

Reporting in the September 21, 2007 issue of the journal Cell, researcher David Sinclair from Harvard Medical School, in collaboration with scientists from Cornell Medical School and the National Institutes of Health, discovered two additional genes in mammalian cells that act as gatekeepers for cellular longevity. When cells experience certain kinds of stress, such as caloric restriction, these genes rev up and help protect cells from diseases of aging.

The new genes discovered are called *SIRT-3* and *SIRT-4*. Like SIRT-1, they are part of the larger class of sirtuins. The newly discovered role of SIRT-3 and SIRT-4 confirmed the particular importance of mitochondria as vital for sustaining the health and longevity of a cell.

Mitochondria, a kind of "cellular organ" that lives in the cytoplasm, are often considered to be the cell's battery packs or energy producing factories. When mitochondria become compromised by particular stressors, energy is drained out of the cell, and its days are numbered. This, in turn compromises our energy production, health and metabolic efficiency. Sinclair and his colleagues discovered that

SIRT-3 and SIRT-4 play a vital role in a longevity network that maintains the vitality of mitochondria and keeps cells healthy when they would otherwise die. The most powerful method found of activating these life saving/life-extending genes is caloric restriction.

When cells undergo caloric restriction, signals sent in through the membrane activate a gene called NAMPT. As levels of NAMPT ramp up, a small molecule called NAD begins to amass in the mitochondria. This, in turn, causes the activity of enzymes created by the SIRT-3 and SIRT-4 genes—enzymes that live in the mitochondria—to increase as well. As a result, the mitochondria grow stronger, energy-output increases, and the cell's aging process slows down significantly.

In laboratory experiments certain animal subjects have been able to extend their healthy life spans by 30–60%—even up to 300–400%—using methods of optimal caloric restriction! The implications are staggering. The same basic mechanism seems to exist across all species studied, from yeast to even primates.

But *why* does caloric restriction work?

Why would mimicking starvation have such a profound effect on extending life span? It almost seems counter-intuitive. The answer to this mysterious question had been the Holy Grail of longevity researchers for close to seventy-five years.

Now we know.

In the early 1990s, there was an unusual discovery made by a researcher, Cynthia Kenyon, PhD, Professor of Biochemistry and Biophysics at the University of California, San Francisco. She was studying an ancient species of worm (a nematode called *C. elegans*). This particular little worm—from a species that has been around for millions and millions of years—developed a genetic mutation that, quite unusually, seemed to more than double the worm's life span—the most significant life extension that had been reported in any organism up to that point. In 1993, Dr. Kenyon and colleagues published a study in *Nature* that describes this life-extending genetic mutation. Normally, mutations are not considered to be a particularly beneficial thing—they typically are more inclined to kill or greatly inconvenience an organism.

This was different. They called this mysterious, magical mutated gene the *DAF-2* gene.

A few years later, the research team actually discovered what this gene did. It rocked the entire scientific world in the field of longevity research. They'd found their Holy Grail. *The DAF-2 gene essentially encoded an insulin receptor.* In other words, when insulin was down-regulated in this worm, the worm lived longer. *Much* longer.

Since when does something like a worm produce insulin, you ask? Insulin in these simple life forms has nothing to do with blood sugar regulation, but instead is entirely designed to regulate reproduction and actual life span. Subsequent research has confirmed this role of insulin across all species, including primates:

How much insulin we produce over the course of our lives literally controls how long we live! And it turns out the less insulin needed—the better.

Studies looking at the effects of insulin levels on human health and longevity are emerging, and the picture is quite clear. One study showed that over a ten-year period, the risk of dying was almost twice as great for those with the highest insulin levels than for those with the lowest levels. The study authors stated that excess insulin, or hyperinsulinemia, is associated with increased all-cause and cardiovascular mortality independent of other risk factors (Dekker, et al, 2005). High- serum insulin promotes high blood pressure by impairing sodium balance. Prolonged exposure to excess insulin can severely compromise the vascular system. By acting as a catalyst in promoting cellular proliferation, excess insulin also increases the risk for and progression of certain cancers. High insulin promotes the formation of beta-amyloid in brain cells and may contribute to the development of Alzheimer's disease. Overproduction of insulin even contributes to prostate enlargement by helping to promote the overgrowth of prostate cells. Insulin resistance, a by-product of chronic excess insulin production, is associated with the development of abdominal obesity and health problems such as atherosclerosis and impotence. Furthermore, insulin resistance and obesity are risk factors for type 2 diabetes. Hyperinsulinemia is predictive for type 2 diabetes mellitus.

It turns out that insulin is an extremely ancient molecule and exists in identical form, in everything from yeast cells to humans. Far from the formerly perceived limited role in nutrient storage or even "blood sugar control" (a trivial sideline for insulin), insulin is now being understood as something far more important and fundamental to the very underlying mechanisms of our health and longevity. In monitoring our energy availability, while leptin oversees the actual energy stores it is insulin that switches on and off the extremely ancient mechanisms that allow us to outlive an apparent famine.

That's the clue to as to how we beat Nature at her own game. The down-regulation of insulin (and mTOR) triggers the up-regulation of repair and maintenance on a cellular level that allows us to remain healthy until food becomes more available and we can "finally reproduce."

That's our magic "loophole."

What do all the longest-living individuals have in common?

"If there is a known single marker for long life, as found in the centenarian and animal studies, it is low insulin levels."
—RON ROSEDALE, MD, 1998

Research across the board has shown that long-lived individuals (animals and humans) share the following characteristics:

- Low fasting insulin levels
- Low fasting glucose
- Optimally low leptin
- Low triglycerides
- Low percentage of visceral body fat
- Lower body temperature
- Reduced thyroid levels

Low thyroid, you say? Isn't that a bad thing?

The idea here is that a reduced caloric load, the almost entirely exclusive use of fat for fuel and optimal nutrient intake, improves metabolic *efficiency*. As long as things are operating efficiently, higher metabolism isn't necessary or even desirable. Your internal engine runs less hot, and the engine therefore lasts longer.

This isn't to say that having low thyroid in a blood chemistry or salivary hormone panel is always necessarily good at all. It's a contextual thing. If your thyroid is low because you've been burning your adrenals out, or because you've developed Hashimoto's autoimmune disease and are producing thyroid peroxidase (TPO) antibodies, that's not so good. It's all relative. The *reason* why your thyroid is low is more important than the condition in and of itself.

In a person, however, that has the rest of the above laboratory markers, a low level of T4 (thyroxin) may be perfectly acceptable . . . even desirable!

One single longevity marker stands out among all long-lived animals and persons above the rest, however, and that's *low insulin levels*.

USING INSULIN AND LEPTIN
TO OUR ADVANTAGE

It remains true that leptin actually is what controls the bigger hormonal picture in humans (and other mammals). When leptin levels repeatedly surge in response to dietary elevations of starch or sugar this has a numbing effect on the ability of our hypothalamus to "hear" leptin's message. We become leptin resistant. The brain effectively stops hearing leptin's message and assumes its levels are too low, and that we are starving—even though the image you see in your mirror tells a different story. This, in turn, compels our hypothalamus send out a direct signal to eat more and tells insulin to increase and store more fat.

When leptin levels are optimally low, however, and our taste for fat is satisfied, insulin signaling also quiets—fat burning, repair, regeneration and maintenance are up-regulated, instead—effectively increasing our health and individual lifespan.

How do we control leptin to our advantage? By eating just enough dietary fat, *in the absence of carbohydrate* (and other insulin generating stimuli, including excess protein), to satisfy our appetite and assure our hypothalamus that "hunting is good."

Since leptin controls hunger and leptin is the primary sensor for fat, and since we are creatures of the Ice Age for whom fat basically means survival, eating fat as our dominant source of fuel—the way we were actually designed—is our ultimate key to the mystery of health and long-term survival.

We don't need genetic manipulation or new longevity drugs. We can do it all with diet, easily, inexpensively and simply.

By eliminating unnecessary carbohydrates (basically, all dietary sugar and starch) and effectively minimizing insulin, by consuming *just enough* protein to meet our basic maintenance and repair requirements and keeping mTOR down-regulated, by "feeding our hypothalamus" via healthy leptin signaling, and by feeding our cells with the fat and fat soluble nutrients that nourish and supply us with long, even-burning, non-glycating, satisfying energy—we can enjoy a level of health and vitality one might never have believed was possible.

It is all actually very simple. Using these exact same principles and controlling these same primal mechanisms, it may be possible to halt or even reverse many of the disease processes we have come to associate with aging, including cancer. A body focused entirely on its own repair, healing, regeneration and maintenance will enjoy powerfully enhanced immune function, energy, and well-being—even reversing many of the signs and symptoms of aging.

How cool is that?

Is there any other way?

Certain newly discovered nutrients such as *trans-resveratrol* (found in grape skins) have been shown to also have an activating effect on sirtuins, particularly SIRT-1. *Trans*-resveratrol, the only active form of resveratrol, has been shown to increase immunity, control blood pressure, preserve red blood cells, inhibit fungal infection, protect the liver and the heart, improve insulin sensitivity, prevent blood clots and inhibit inflammation. Studies suggest it could be a cure for cancer, heart disease and age-related brain disorders among scores of other things. Some scientists feel trans-resveratrol could even help extend human lifespan up to 70% (or up to 50 years). It's pretty exciting stuff.

Resveratrol is found in minute amounts in red wine and is produced by a variety of plants when put under stress. In 2003, it was first discovered and reported in *Nature* to have anti-aging properties by David Sinclair and Joseph Baur, other Harvard Medical School researchers, and their colleagues. This has resulted in the media and press promoting red wine as though it were the ultimate fountain of youth in a bottle. To match the benefits of resveratrol found in studies with mice, however, the average human would have to drink roughly a hundred glasses or more of wine to obtain a similarly beneficial daily dose. (Oh, well, off to happy hour we go . . .)

Caveat emptor: Most commercial supplements sold as "resveratrol" contain only, or mostly, the *cis*-form, which is largely inactive. *Trans*-resveratrol, the only active form, though available in some supplements, needs to be taken in relatively high doses—some researchers estimate the beneficial dose needed to mimic caloric restriction effects in humans is likely close to 100 mg or possibly more per day. This can be extremely expensive. Prepare to pay $75–$150 a month or more for the "real thing." Also, beware of rip-offs. Many supplement companies will jump on this bandwagon, and only very few—mainly "healthcare practitioner brands"—will deliver the real deal . . . at a substantial price.

Thus far, the best proven and easiest tool most of us have to reverse many signs of aging and extend quality and quantity of life is in the minimization of insulin by minimizing insulin-provoking foods and substances—plus moderating a quality protein intake. The modified version of caloric restriction presented in this book can work for anyone, and far more affordably and sustainably than other dietary approaches. For those who can afford it, though, the addition of trans-resveratrol to this dietary approach could have some pretty exciting implications.

PART TWO:
PRIMAL MIND

Your body IS your subconscious mind!
—CANDACE PERT, PhD

THE CONNECTION BETWEEN DIET, NUTRIENT DEFICIENCIES AND MOOD DISORDERS, ATTENTIONAL PROBLEMS, COGNITIVE FUNCTION AND WELL-BEING

The myth, of course, is to suppose that there is a real distinction between body and mind. There is, in fact, no fundamental separation between mind and body. What happens to one happens to the other. They are both part of the same functioning or dysfunctioning system and must be understood together in context. The best psychotherapy, brain training or medication cannot put a nutrient there that is not there, or remove some damaging substance that doesn't belong. It cannot even begin to compensate for poor dietary tendencies.

The brain and body need certain raw materials in order to function—*period*. Without proper and sufficient raw materials (i.e., proper nutrition), no amount of any quality therapy or intervention will ever have optimal or lasting results. Toxic stressors, be they sugar or starch, alcohol, heavy metals, excitotoxins, xenoestrogens, contaminants or EMF pollution, cannot be overridden with any amount of psychotherapy, or the addition of more toxic stressors in the form of prescription drugs. Furthermore, *all* neurotransmitters and neuropeptides have receptors that exist in literally every organ and system in the body. Of the nearly three hundred internal communication substances, nearly all are shared throughout the entire body and are anything but unique to the brain. Nor are even neurons unique to the brain; they exist abundantly elsewhere in the body.

The mind (including memory and emotion) is not simply contained in the brain . . . it exists as a "field" throughout the entire human organism! What is done to the mind is done to the body . . . and vice versa. You simply cannot separate the two.

Prozac Nation

In 1985, the total annual sales for all antidepressants in the United States were approximately $240 million. Today, it is in excess of $12 *billion*. Between 1987 and 1997, the percentage of Americans in outpatient treatment for depression more than tripled. Of those in treatment, the percentage of prescribed medication nearly doubled. Of the three hundred most commonly prescribed medications, *none actually serve to support natural physiological functioning*.

Medications artificially manipulate biochemistry in an effort to ameliorate symptoms. All possess the potential for side effects and endocrine disruption. Exacerbation of nutrient deficiencies and endocrine disruption occur to some degree with most, if not all drugs.

The fact is, all psychoactive drugs act upon cellular receptors that are designed for our own naturally produced counterparts. The very use of these psychoactive drugs can diminish the sensitivity to our own endogenously made chemicals over time and disrupt healthy cellular communication and functioning, ultimately making matters worse, long term (even when there seems to be short-term benefit). Nutritional and dietary imbalances, food sensitivities, toxic influences and neurological timing issues may affect virtually every disorder. There are natural solutions to virtually everything, as the human body and brain are miraculously equipped to heal themselves if facilitated by the presence of needed raw materials, liberation from toxic burdens and an appropriate, healthy attitude.

It takes a certain determination and willingness to take responsibility for one's own well-being. It takes a certain decision to take charge of discovering the answers for one's self. Sometimes (in keeping with human nature), it takes reaching the point where the pain of the problem is worse than the pain of the long-term solution, to arrive at real lasting change. Health is a choice we all make and a responsibility we ourselves shoulder. No magic pill will ever take the place of a diet and lifestyle that honors our primal physiology.

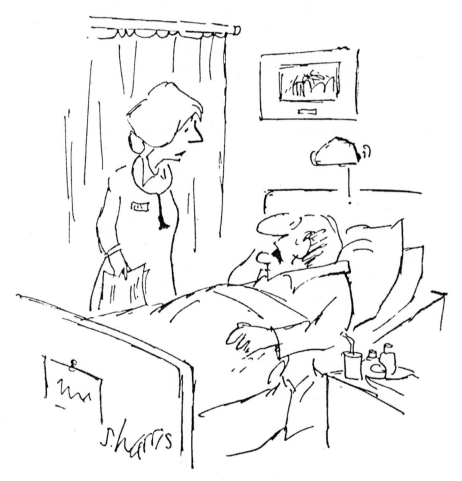

"I STOPPED TAKING THE MEDICINE BECAUSE I PREFER THE ORIGINAL DISEASE TO THE SIDE EFFECTS."

My own clinical experience

As a clinical Neurofeedback Specialist, my orientation is to approach the symptoms of cognitive and emotional dysregulation as, to some degree, dysregulations of arousal (together with improper neurological "communication," phase relationships and bio-electric timing mechanisms). Contrary to the ever-thickening *Diagnostic and Statistical Manual of Mental Disorders* (DSM-IV), the neurofeedback approach is infinitely simple by comparison. A nervous system may be functionally "under-aroused," "over-aroused," some combination thereof, or is in a state of "unstable arousal," combined with either or both under- and over-arousal.

Training is approached, at least initially, from one of these standpoints. (Of course, I'm over simplifying a bit.)

Most presenting symptoms fall into one of these related categories. The vast majority of clients that *I* see nowadays can readily be categorized as cases of either over-arousal or unstable arousal. This has become increasingly the case over time in recent years. Training helps restore healthy communication and the brain essentially learns to regulate itself.

By far, the single greatest influence mitigating these forms of dysregulation I see every day is diet . . . and, to the point, specifically blood sugar dysregulation together with insulin and leptin resistance. Food sensitivities and deficiencies are also extremely common, and endemic mainly to carbohydrate-based diets, as well. Nothing can serve to compromise anything and everything to do with brain function or get in the way of restoration of healthy brain function more than a lousy diet. What are the implications?

Everything you have ever experienced, felt, or conducted in life is due to brain function. The ability to enjoy, perceive, sense, and experience life is dictated by the firing rate and health of your brain. It is impossible for a person to become healthy mentally or physiologically without a healthy brain.

—DATIS KHARRAZIAN, DC, DHSc, MS, MNeuroSci(c), FAACP, DACBN, DIBAK, CNS, CCN, CSCS, CCSP, 2008

Far and away, the most damaged and intractably dysregulated brains and nervous systems I have seen or dealt with in my practice have all essentially been vegans, with strict vegetarians a close second—*hands down*. I have numerous other colleagues who have made the same independent observation. A diet of starch, sugar, lectins, phytates and common allergens, or food-sensitivity-generating foods, coupled with chronic deficiencies: of numerous critical essential fats (EPA/DHA, healthy saturates), fat soluble nutrients (preformed A, D, E and K), amino-acid imbalances and/or deficiencies and other key animal source nutrients—not the least of which is utilizable B12 (and B12 analogs from seaweed don't count)—lead to states of over-arousal, anxiety-related disorders, memory problems, cognitive dysfunction, sleep disturbances, brain degeneration, GI disorders and utter metabolic chaos. It is deeply problematic. These unnaturally restrictive diets, **together with other carbohydrate-based diets** dysregulate insulin and leptin function to the extreme.

Remember that the hormone leptin controls virtually all functions of the hypothalamus. That's a lot of control.

These issues concerning carbohydrate excesses, more than any other, underlie to some degree most of what I see as mood or behavioral issues, as well as a whole lot of other things, and at least plays *some* role in all of it.

It is well-established that elevated insulin and leptin both generate and exacerbate sympathetic over-arousal ("fight or flight" mode).

Surges of these hormones, mainly driven by chronic excess carbohydrate consumption, are both anxiety-provoking and destabilizing to the nervous system. Diets lacking in adequate quality fat are further destabilizing. It is a vicious, often self-perpetuating cycle. Neurofeedback can accomplish an incredible amount of progress with an individual all on its own, powerfully raising the internal "stress-threshold" and training self-regulation, but the combination of effective dietary measures with quality brain training is both synergistic *and* profound. I see this every day.

How we get there in the first place

Simply put, stress and trauma (whether physical, emotional or biochemical), basically shove us off whatever cliff we happen to be standing next to. Wherever our vulnerability lies, in both our inherent makeup and with our current state of health—that is the direction we go. The brain's timing mechanisms and phase relationships can become functionally deranged and help kindle certain tendencies at these points of vulnerability. Some people, when "shoved," fall into a perpetual state of anxiety . . . others depression, or bipolar disorder, or migraines, or seizures, or addiction, etc. It's a long list. We are all individuals and no two respond exactly the same, to any given stimuli or trauma.

We see the world around us through the lens of our hormones, neurotransmitters and, to the degree which we are dependent upon it, blood sugar. Unhealthy hormonal patterns generate unhealthy arousal patterns and, consequently, unhealthy emotional and behavioral tendencies. We wake up with "low blood sugar" due to insulin dysregulation and poor diet, and we feel lousy. We then proceed to interpret the lousy feeling through associating it with events and people in our lives, assuming they are to blame (and that life simply sucks), rather than recognizing that we are operating under distorted, biochemically-induced misperceptions. We become "hijacked" by our dysregulated nervous systems, behave in ways we abhor and may even feel we are somehow fundamentally "flawed" as a person because of it. This is a *huge* source of self-esteem problems. We then continue to interpret the world around us through this warped lens and beat ourselves up for our own short-comings.

At any given moment, we all have positive things in our lives and challenging things we could be focused on as our reality. Why do we gravitate toward focusing on one thing versus another? *The functioning of our hormones—specifically insulin and leptin—to a very large extent, influences the way we focus on and interpret the world around us and the events in our lives.* The secondary effects of blood sugar, insulin and leptin dysregulation, which are a part of this, involve the disruption and depletion of neurotransmitter functioning. It is a huge issue and profoundly influences the way many interpret and respond—or react to their world. Is it any wonder why our society is in such a state of chaos?

Nothing will ever influence the functioning or dysfunctioning of your hormones or neurotransmitters (or your brain) more than the issue of blood sugar. Where neurotransmitters are concerned—our main mood and brain regulators, surges of blood sugar generate surges, and subsequent depletion and/or dysregulation, of serotonin, epinephrine, norepinephrine, gamma-aminobutyric acid (GABA) and dopamine. Blood sugar surges also deplete B-complex needed for the manufacture of neurotransmitters, along with an additional few hundred other things; and magnesium, needed for parasympathetic (relaxed) functioning, liver detoxification, DHA synthesis and another few hundred other things.

Eating foods to which one is sensitive stimulates surges in cortisol or stress hormones, and, subsequently, insulin, as well as histamine, which acts as an excitatory neurotransmitter and can agitate the nervous system. Insulin surges actually prevent the movement of L-tryptophan across the blood-brain barrier and block most all other neurotransmitter function. A brain that is dependent on glucose for its functioning will experience considerable compromise during these fluctuations—and moods, together with cognitive functioning, will tend to be unstable and/or at the mercy of blood sugar availability. A brain functioning instead on ketones, of course, would have no such vulnerability (though food sensitivities still need to be monitored and deficiencies addressed).

Blood sugar surges stimulate accelerated glycation, insulin, leptin, inflammatory cytokines and cortisol—which collectively contribute to the degeneration of the brain and its functioning *more than any other factor,* as well as being significantly disruptive to numerous bodily processes. The brain is enormously vulnerable to the glycating ravages (AGEs) of glucose, attracting aggressive oxidative processes, further degrading its delicate structure and diminishing functional capacity. The more the brain degenerates, the more prone to chronic neurological sympathetic over-arousal the brain becomes. Anxiety and anxiety-related disorders today are utterly epidemic.

By optimizing our dietary choices and our brains, and minimizing our dependence upon glucose for fuel, we alter the framework of our entire lives. It's more than just being about "staying healthy" . . . it's about positively re-shaping our internal experience toward what it literally means to be alive.

What could possibly be more important?

THE BIOLOGY OF BELIEF:
THE REAL "SECRET"

There is a great deal of attention being given today to the New Age concept that "belief" drives our reality, our biology and our health. There is some real scientific validity to this, in fact, though forcing oneself to "think positive thoughts," while simultaneously suppressing or sublimating what one is actually feeling inside is not necessarily the fast track to better mental (or physical) health. If anything, it's likely to make things worse. Cultivating *authenticity* to one's experience of emotions—being more fully aware and experiencing them for what they really are, *then* asking oneself constructive questions about how to best and most positively approach any given situation is far more productive. Additionally, learning to effectively release negative thoughts and feelings is actually much easier and more natural than trying to force positive thinking (check out *The Sedona Method*).

"New Age guilt" is rampant—feeling somehow responsible for your own illness or tragedy in life and beating yourself up because you "harbored negative thoughts" is a pointless pastime. **If there is one single belief that people should cultivate, however, it's that we are ultimately responsible for our own health—and it is up to us to take that responsibility seriously and not simply entrust it to others who claim to have the answers and have their own agenda.**

> No one will ever be more invested in your mental or physical health than you.

It has never been more important for us all to fundamentally understand how our bodies and minds work, and *never more important to take our diets and stress management seriously.* Take charge of your own mental, emotional and physical health and recognize that anything is possible!

Given the appropriate raw materials (diet) and a removal of toxic burdens and unhealthy lifestyle factors, positive thinking and feeling becomes a *natural state* that doesn't need to be artificially cultivated. It simply flows.

It's our primal birthright.

HOW IMPORTANT IS FAT
TO THE BRAIN?

The brain is our single most expensive organ, with respect to metabolic needs in the body. It occupies only 5% of our total mass, but it literally utilizes at least 20% or more of our body's energy supply to meet its considerable demands. Many people assume that the brain needs glucose for this energy, but few are aware that the brain actually prefers ketones, the energy units of fat, for its dominant source of fuel!

The brain can and does use glucose, especially when a person consumes a diet that is dominated by carbohydrates or during an emergency, though glucose isn't as essential to the day-to-day functioning of the brain as it is commonly presented or believed. In the absence of carbohydrates, once metabolically adapted, the brain will readily and naturally turn to ketones for its primary source of fuel.

The brain uses ketones in a state of ketosis. Cerebral ketone utilization is prevalent, for instance, in newborn infants nursing on fat-rich mother's milk. The switch to dependence on glucose does not occur until carbohydrates are introduced into the child's diet. The enzymes responsible for ketone metabolism, *d-β-hydroxybutyrate dehydrogenase, acetoacetate-succinyl-CoA transferase,* and *acetoacetyl-CoA-thiolase,* are present in brain tissue in sufficient amounts to convert them into acyl-CoA and to feed them into the tricarboxylic acid cycle at a sufficient rate to satisfy the metabolic demands of the brain (*Basic Neurochemistry*, 1999). Cerebral utilization of ketones is increased more or less in direct proportion to the degree of ketosis.

The body preferentially burns excess sugar whenever it is present, mainly to rid the body of this damaging substance any way it can. Sugar or glucose will also dominate as a source of brain fuel where turbo-charged energy is in sudden demand, such as in an emergency. Sufficient carbohydrate stores in the form of glycogen in the liver are always available for this.

Depending entirely upon glucose as a primary fuel for the brain and body is ultimately unnatural, however, and problematic—and this is the metabolic state in which the vast majority of people reside. Brain cells don't respond much to insulin and are therefore more vulnerable than just about any other tissue to the ravages of glycation and the oxidation or free radical activity that glucose and glycation attracts. There is no such thing as a "safe" low level of glucose. Glucose and other sugars, such as fructose, always glycate us and attract free radical activity, to some ongoing degree, no matter what. Although we need glucose to some extent for feeding our red blood cells, glucose is really what eventually kills many of us—a cruel irony. We do maintain some control over the rate of glycation and degeneration, though, through what we choose to eat and what supplements we take.

Glycation is the primary cause of brain degeneration in aging and also of Alzheimer's. (Alzheimer's is basically a state of brain neuropathy. Notice the sweet tooth in many Alzheimer's patients.) Beta-amyloid proteins, or glycated tangles of proteins, clump and stick together in the brain and eventually cause the symptoms later identified as Alzheimer's disease. The same sort of damage that is done to the brain in alcoholism occurs at a slow, but steady rate when consuming any form of a carbohydrate-, sugar- and/or starch-rich diet.

When the brain and body learn, instead, to burn ketones as their primary source of fuel, the brain is spared much of this damage and is fed with a far more sustainable, reliable and abundant source of energy to meet its constant metabolic needs. One is far less subject to "blood sugar lows" and the mental, emotional and physical symptoms associated with it. Blood sugar is thus essentially eliminated from the mood and cognitive equation. The utilization of anti-glycating nutrients can further protect from and help reverse, to at least some degree, these degenerative processes.

So . . . How important is fat to the health of the brain?

Immeasurably.

The brain is made up of more than 50% fat—up to 70–80% of dry weight. In fact, the body's highest concentrations of omega-3 fatty acids are in the brain; up to one quarter of the human brain's fatty acid stores are DHA—a component of omega-3s commonly found in cold-water fish oils and meats of exclusively pasture-fed animals or wild game. Humans are unique among primates, in this regard; the brains of chimps and other primates are dominated by omega-6s. Omega-3s, conversely, are entirely essential—*vital*—to the normal electrical functioning, as well as cardiovascular, joint, immune and gastrointestinal health of the human brain and nervous system. Omega-3s are utterly vital for proper and efficient intercellular communication and anti-inflammatory processes. The consumption of utilizable carbohydrates, however, and elevated insulin, disrupts omega-3 metabolism and causes the kidneys to dump magnesium—a mineral absolutely needed for the conversion of EPA to DHA, the storage molecule of omega-3 in the brain and vital to all functions there. Insulin also tends to divert prostaglandin production to more pro-inflammatory omega-6 pathways.

As much as 10% of human brain size has been lost in just the last century alone, likely due to decreased amounts of available dietary EPA and DHA and increased consumption of processed foods (Leonard, et al).

The loss of magnesium through blood sugar surges, together with the absence of adequate dietary magnesium (and/or poor HCL production and digestion) also allows for the binding of structurally related but toxic elements, such as aluminum and others to its vacant receptor sites. Elevated aluminum levels in the brain, of course, have also been associated with Alzheimer's disease. Magnesium, in addition, controls over three hundred enzymes in the body and mind, is critical for maintaining healthy parasympathetic functioning—a calm, relaxed nervous system—and is commonly deficient in those consuming a higher carbohydrate diet.

Omega-3s may be the single most commonly deficient nutrient in the modern human—particularly Western—diet. Supplementation with fish oils today provides the most reliable and affordable sources of both EPA and DHA, omega-3's most important derivatives. Antarctic krill oil is another potentially even more highly effective, though much more expensive source of EPA/DHA. Antarctic krill oil contains unique phospholipids and antioxidants not present in fish oil that may better facilitate its absorption, preservation and utilization, and can be a viable alternative to fish oil for some who are willing to pay significantly more. Our ancestors got preformed EPA and DHA by consuming high quantities of naturally and exclusively grass-fed wild game, organ meats and wild-caught cold-water fish, where available.

Over-cooking rapidly denatures and destroys these oils, as they are highly polyunsaturated.

Deficiencies of omega-3s are often particularly pronounced in those with depression, insulin resistance, obesity, bipolar illness, cardiovascular disease and ADD/HD, and supplementation has been shown at times to markedly benefit these conditions. *Fish oils are overwhelmingly preferable to flax oil,* as many individuals with learning disabilities and other mental/emotional/cognitive disorders are known to lack the delta-6 desaturase enzyme necessary to create EPA and DHA from the "parent" form of omega-3 in vegetable sources, alpha-linolenic acid (ALA). A mere 3–5% or less of ALA (in flax oil, walnuts, etc) ever makes it to becoming EPA. Even less becomes the brain's vitally needed form, DHA (Enig, 2002).

It is also known that trans fats in the body interfere with this metabolic pathway, as does magnesium deficiency, excess amounts of omega-6 (corn, sunflower, safflower . . . etc.), which compete for these enzymes biochemically.

The over consumption of vegetable oils—such as soy and canola (which are usually partially hydrogenated), safflower, sunflower and corn oils (omega-6), cottonseed oil (extremely high in pro-inflammatory omega-6 and not even a food-source oil), margarines or vegetable shortenings, which contain hydrogenated trans fats, and even excess olive oil (omega-9) can interfere with the body's utilization of omega-3s. These exacerbate insulin resistance—leading to obesity, atherosclerosis, etc.—and cause mutagenic changes leading to numerous cancers. With the exception of olive oil, these vegetable oils are best avoided entirely. Olive oil is okay for salads, over steamed vegetables, or as an accent to various dishes, though I don't advise over-using it or actually cooking with it as it can easily rancidify when exposed to higher heat.

Hydrogenated and partially hydrogenated fats should never be used at all. Ever. Don't be fooled by claims of "reduced trans fats" in fast foods or processed food items, or by packaging that claims "zero trans fat," then lists soybean oil, regular, non-organic canola oil, or any other partially hydrogenated ingredient. Labeling laws currently allow a certain amount of trans fat per serving before it has to be disclosed. The food industry takes advantage of labeling loopholes everywhere it can. The more one can simply avoid processed or packaged products, the better.

The only safe amount of trans fat is zero.

Naturally occurring saturated fat and cholesterol do not compete with omega-3s, and, in fact, are mutually beneficial physiologically. In addition, saturated fat and cholesterol, unjustly vilified, provide both cell membrane integrity and *resistance to oxidation,* and make up at least 50% of cell membranes. Naturally occurring saturated fat also assists in absorption of vital nutrients, plays a vital role in bone modeling, lowers Lipoprotein(a), a marker for heart disease, protects the liver from alcohol ingestion, enhances the immune system, is needed for the proper utilization of essential fatty acids, energy production, normal hormonal production and normal cellular metabolism. Shorter-chain saturated fatty acids (3–14 carbons in length) have potent antimicrobial and antiviral properties as well (Enig).

"It would seem that our glands effect control far above proportion to their size, and this is true. It is also true, however, that the glands have their master, probably the most remarkable creation in all of life's miracles—the human brain."

—Dr. Bernard Jensen, PhD

WHERE DOES ADD/HD
FIT IN TO ALL OF THIS?

There is some inexplicably lingering, weak debate among scientists as to the effect of dietary sugar and carbohydrates on behavior in children. But sugar—and some other high-glycemic foods, as well as artificial counterparts such as aspartame (Nutrasweet) and sucrolose (Splenda)—enters the bloodstream quickly and has commonly been reported to induce hyperactivity and other behavioral problems in children (*New England Journal of Medicine,* 1994).

Other high-glycemic and insulin-generating foods, in addition to simple or refined sugars, include such things as: pasta, noodles, breads (whole grain or otherwise), rice, and potatoes, together with other starchy vegetables. The consumption of high-glycemic foods, which cause a rapid rise in blood sugar, can trigger many behavioral, learning and mood problems. When a child or adult is glucose dependent and does not eat frequently enough, eats foods to which he or she may be sensitive/allergic, or has a diet that is high in carbohydrate-rich foods, blood sugar levels can rise and drop dramatically. To pull these levels back to normal, the body releases adrenaline. Adrenaline triggers sympathetic nervous system activity: basically the "fight or flight" response. It can be good to have high adrenaline levels if one's life is in immediate danger (that's what adrenaline is for), but it is extremely difficult to sit, listen and behave when adrenaline release occurs while in the classroom (Block, 1997), D.O., Mary Ann—"Treating Attention Deficit Disorder Naturally"—*Nature's Impact, October/November 1997*).

Avoiding excess carbohydrates is obviously key, as is the regular consumption of protein- and fat-rich foods throughout the day. Protein and fat consumption normalizes blood sugar and also provides a vital source of amino acids and other key fat-soluble nutrients for normal and stable neurological functioning.

Essential fatty acids (EFAs), particularly in the form of omega-3, are known to be widely deficient in the modern diet and *especially* in those who manifest cognitive or affective disorders, ADD and other learning disabilities.

Ultra-prevalent trans fats found in most processed foods cereals, salad dressings, condiments, snacks, commercial vegetable oils, breads and fast-foods—in many cases constituting up to 20% of daily caloric intake—interfere with absorption and utilization of all essential fatty acids and lead to additional cognitive impairment, inflammation and disease. *Elimination of these unnatural fats from the diet is essential.* Elimination from the body once ingested and incorporated into one's cellular structure, however, may take time—*up to two years* (Enig, 2002).

Read all labels carefully. When in restaurants, always ask what fats are being used in cooking and salad dressings. Restaurant owners need to be made aware this stuff matters, too!

Other foods commonly reported to cause problems include conventionally-produced milk and chicken eggs, chocolate, soy, wheat, corn, and peanuts. Also included as problematic are preservatives, artificial colors, pesticides and other synthetic compounds found in processed foods. A paleolithically-oriented diet would be naturally free (mostly) of such dietary inclusions. All of these foods may be considered fairly recent (i.e., 10,000 years ago or less) additions to the human diet. Of these, the one most commonly associated with ADHD is clearly gluten sensitivity. Some estimate that 70–80% of all ADHD cases are gluten sensitive individuals, commonly advanced to celiac disease. A study done in 2006 stated in conclusion: "The data indicate that ADHD-like symptomatology is markedly overrepresented among untreated Celiac Disease (CD) patients and that a gluten-free diet may improve symptoms significantly within a short period of time. The results of this study also suggest that CD should be included in the list of diseases associated with ADHD-like symptomatology." (J Atten Disord 2006 Nov;10(2):200–4).

A protein called *zonulin* has recently been discovered in elevated levels in individuals with ADHD, as well as autism, MS and numerous psychiatric disorders. Zonulin is known to regulate intestinal permeability and is known to be associated with celiac disease. Tissue samples from symptomatic celiac patients had higher levels of zonulin and anti-zonulin antibodies than samples either from patients on gluten-free diets or those without the disease. "People with celiac have an increased level of zonulin, which opens the junctions between the cells. In essence, the gateways are stuck open, allowing gluten and other allergens to pass [through]," according to Alessio Fasano, professor of pediatrics and physiology at the University of Maryland School of Medicine. "Once these allergens get into the immune system, they are attacked by the antibodies." *(Applied Genetics News, May, 2000).*

Researchers believe that the higher levels of zonulin may explain how a molecule as large as gluten can cross the intestinal wall and incite the creation of antibodies. Zonulin also helps regulate the permeability of the blood-brain barrier and could be a factor in other autoimmune diseases. The implications of this are very serious and can only be remedied by a strict adherence to a gluten-free diet. One can test for gluten sensitivity, as well as sensitivity to casein, soy and eggs via EnteroLab using a stool antigen test anyone can order. (www. enterolab.com)

In an open study of 78 children with ADHD referred to a nutrition clinic, 59 improved on a few foods trial that eliminated foods to which children are commonly sensitive; for the 19 children in this study who were able to participate in a double-blind cross-over trial of the suspected food, there was a significant effect for the provoking foods to worsen ratings of behavior and to impair psychological test performance. (*Lifestyle and Complementary Therapies for ADHD: How Health Professionals Can Approach Patients*—Medscape 2007). Food sensitivities must always be considered in addressing ADHD symptoms.

Other dietary considerations:

Supplementation with fish oils in small quantities—only 1–2% of caloric intake—not only enhances the functioning of the brain and nervous system, as well as cardiovascular and immune systems, but also tends to help eliminate unhealthy cravings for sweets, once adequate protein and deficient EFA levels are replenished.

Remember: If EPA and DHA aren't in your diet, then they're not in your brain! It is also critical to note that saturated fat is an essential factor in the protection, transport and utilization of these important and fragile oils and should not be overly restricted in the diet, particularly in children. Cholesterol, too, is utterly vital to the neurological functioning of children and adults alike.

B-complex, in general, is especially important for cognitive functioning and is readily depleted with carbohydrate consumption. Methyl donors such as B6, B12 and folic acid—as well as betaine, s-adenosyl methionine (SAMe), dimethylglycine (DMG), trimethylglgycine (TMG)—are especially important for healthy brain function and metabolism. Regular use of a sublingual methylcobalamin B12 supplement can be especially helpful, in this regard. B12 may be less well absorbed from food, or even in pill or capsule forms by many with compromised digestion. There is no toxicity associated with B12.

A more recently recognized and tragically overlooked factor in many cases of ADHD involves **iodine deficiency**. Iodine is needed and utilized by each and every cell in the body. It can make for a night and day difference in many cases of ADHD and is a likely deficiency in most cases of the disorder. It is also needed for the proper functioning of each and every single hormone, to say nothing of normal thyroid function. The absence of iodine in most of our soils and foods today are only part of the problem. The use of "iodized salt" (containing *iodide* and not iodine), useful mainly for minimizing the incidence of goiters (and typically filled with undesirable additives, including aluminum), is poor for providing sufficient tissue levels of **both** forms of iodine needed in the body for optimal functioning.

One study reported in the Journal of Clinical Endocrinology in December of 2004 followed sixteen women who were living in an iodine-deficient area, as well as eleven other women living in an area that was known to be iodine sufficient. In a 10-year follow-up, ADHD had been diagnosed in 11 of the 16 women in the iodine-deficient area vs. ZERO of the eleven in the iodine-sufficient area. Also, IQ was at least 10 points lower in the iodine-deficient area.

The rampant and ubiquitous overuse of halogens such as bromine/bromide, chlorine/chloride and fluorine/fluoride in processed foods, medications, processed vegetable oils, bread, pastas, cereals, pesticides, drinking water and innumerable other daily household items add dramatically to this problem by displacing iodine in our bodies and brains and preventing its absorption. The result to our brains and metabolic functioning is insidiously devastating. I highly recommend carefully reviewing the work of Guy Abraham, MD, FACN and also

David Brownstein, MD for enlightened information on this important topic. I also highly recommend David Brownstein's book: *Iodine: Why You Need It; Why You Can't Live Without It.* Restoring healthy iodine levels is a process that may take several months or even years for some and it should be well and carefully understood. High doses of iodine, particularly when improperly administered can induce uncomfortable detoxification reactions as it displaces toxic halogens and heavy metals, such as mercury, aluminum and arsenic. A gradual building of iodine dosage in a proper and readily utilizable form is very important.

Additionally, certain nutrients such as magnesium, selenium, vitamins E, A, D, B- and C-complex , together with full spectrum (Celtic) sea salt and essential fatty acid (EFA) supplementation are *essential* to iodine absorbing well and being utilized properly in the body. The details are beyond the scope of this book but need to be considered. In the meantime, be sure to include seafood, seaweed and/or kelp supplements as part of your daily diet, as these are among the only reliable food sources of iodine. Kelp and seafood sources tend to be safe and well tolerated by most. Additional iodine supplementation (beyond simply food sources) may be essential for many, however, and I encourage you to seek out a qualified and knowledgeable natural healthcare provider to guide you through the process. The difference appropriate iodine status can make is nothing short of miraculous for those who are deficient (more than 96% of the U.S.) and is well worth the pursuit.

> Important Note: Iodine is needed for the proper metabolism and utilization of dietary cholesterol. Diets higher in cholesterol thereby do utilize and require slightly more iodine.

ADD/HD, LEARNING PROBLEMS, BEHAVIORAL OR MOOD DISORDERS AND THE OMEGA-3 CONNECTION

A Purdue University study showed that kids low in Omega-3 essential fatty acids are significantly more likely to be hyperactive, have learning disorders, and to display behavioral problems. Omega-3 deficiencies have also been tied to dyslexia, violence, depression, memory problems, weight gain, cancer, heart disease, eczema, allergies, inflammatory diseases, arthritis, diabetes and many other conditions.

Over 2000 scientific studies have demonstrated the wide range of problems associated with Omega-3 deficiencies. The American diet is almost devoid of Omega-3s except for certain types of fish. In fact, researchers believe that about 60% of Americans are deficient in Omega-3 fatty acids, and about 20% have so little that test methods cannot even detect any in their blood (Gallagher).

Unfortunately, a significant contributor to the growing trend in these problems in even very young children is *prenatal nutrition*. Children are being born with essential fatty acid (EFA) deficiencies at an alarming rate. Furthermore, no infant formula supplies adequate EPA or DHA, fats so critical to the development of the infant nervous system. Worse yet, soy infant formulas containing phytic acid, trypsin inhibitors and haemagglutinins—not to mention phytoestrogens impacting normal hormonal development—contribute to mineral deficiencies, impacting normal growth and neurological development.

When what little EPA/DHA expectant mothers may have is drained away during pregnancy, postpartum depression is the result. *Expectant mothers have a dramatically increased requirement for EPA and DHA* and should supplement these in the form of molecularly distilled sources of fish oil, as well as with a little cod liver oil to supply critical and commonly deficient fat-soluble nutrients. (Vitamin A is only potentially deleterious during pregnancy in its synthetic forms.)

Trans fats, excessive carbohydrate consumption, processed foods and too many omega-6s in children's diets serve only to severely exacerbate the situation and compound learning and behavior problems. Diets moderately high in quality (read: q-u-a-l-i-t-y) animal source protein—not fast-food burgers and feedlot meat—and sources of omega-3 (from cold-water fish, fish oils and grass-fed meats) are unquestionably vital to a developing young mind and body—and, indeed, to healthy cognitive and physiological functioning at any age.

Memory—*Husker-Du?*

Among the most critical of faculties allowing us to function effectively day to day is basic memory. Memory problems are one of the most common complaints I see and one of the most challenging issues people struggle with. Memory loss is often the result of a progressive degeneration of the brain due to stress/excess cortisol, food sensitivities, glycation and/or environmental factors and is something to be taken very seriously. Certain nutritional deficiencies can also generate or exacerbate this problem.

Perhaps the single most common factor impacting memory function is stress. Our ancestors never could have imagined the degree and sheer volume of chronic stressors on every level most of us experience today. We simply weren't designed for this. Cortisol receptors in the hippocampus (the part of our brain directly over our ears) become over-saturated with this stress hormone and can prompt this part of the brain to start to degenerate. It is no laughing matter when you increasingly forget your words in the middle of a sentence, forget to do everyday things or forget the name of your best friend.

Deficiencies of important fat-soluble nutrients, B vitamins (particularly B12), iodine, zinc, EFA's and other nutrients, take their toll and can accelerate the decline. Chronic sugar or starch consumption is perhaps the single best way to accelerate the problem. Food sensitivities (gluten, casein and others) can set up a vicious never-ending inflammatory response that can degenerate the brain at a record pace, even causing brain lesions.

Pay attention!

Is your memory "not what it used to be?" Please don't ignore the signs. The sooner you take steps to remove antagonistic dietary culprits, replenish depleted nutrients and support healthy regeneration of viable brain tissue, the more likely you may be to stop and even partly reverse the deterioration, and the better the quality of the functioning of your mind and experience of life will be.

So what are some key steps to reclaiming or greatly improving your memory and restoring the health of your brain?

1. Practice stress reduction daily using whatever tools or methods work best for you: meditation, yoga, neurofeedback or biofeedback, heart rate variability training, proper breathing exercises, massage, walking in fresh air—anything. This is not a luxury. It is a necessity.

2. Get six to eight hours of restful sleep each and every single night in a completely dark room.

3. Keep your brain active doing puzzles or simply learning new things. The more you learn, the better you learn!

4. Minimize—or better yet, eliminate—sugar and starch from your diet.

5. Make sure you have adequate essential fatty acids, such as EPA/

DHA (fish oil) and GLA (black currant seed oil) in your diet and avoid low-fat regimens like the plague.

6. Make sure you are properly hydrated. Take your body weight (in pounds), divide by two and this is about the number, in ounces of water your body needs for proper hydration daily. If you drink caffeine, juice or any other diuretic beverage, you should add more water (12–16 oz for every 8 oz of diuretic beverage). Don't exceed a gallon of water per day.

7. Be sure to test for common food sensitivities—particularly gluten and casein—and eliminate foods containing these substances as completely as possible to prevent further damage to your brain and body if they are an issue. (www.enterolab.com)

8. Take a quality phosphorylated or naturally complexed B complex with meals.

9. Minimize the use of cell phones and cordless phones. Scientific evidence is mounting almost exponentially showing evidence of significant brain damage and increased risk for brain lesions and cancers. If you have to use a cell phone, always use the speaker phone option and keep it at least six inches from your head. Headsets (including Bluetooth) can actually make the damage worse.

10. Supplement additionally with *sublingual* B12 in the form of methylcobalamin. It is a key methyl donor in the brain and essential to nervous system health and functioning. This is notoriously (and dangerously) deficient in vegetarians and vegans. Long-term deficiency can result in irreversible neurological damage, memory issues, serious mood and cognitive dysfunction and even dementia-like symptoms. Supplementation is always the safest insurance.

11. Omega-3 fish oil is standard issue for better brain function and cognition, overall. DHA is the most abundant fatty acid in the

human brain . . . however if it isn't in your diet, it isn't in your brain, either! This one is critical and supplementation should be considered.

12. Supplementing with other methyl donors may also be useful, such as: SAMe, DMG, TMG, betaine, choline, B6 and folic acid.

13. Use phosphatidyl serine (PS) to help reverse mild brain degeneration and also help endogenously produce more choline. Research studies showing significant improvement typically utilized 800–2000 mg of phosphatidyl serine per day. PS has been shown to also improve memory, focus and concentration. In research, PS was conjugated with DHA (from fish oils) to optimize utilization, which most available oral PS supplements are not. Transdermal phosphatidyl serine delivery creams (such as AdrenaCalm by Apex Energetics) may be more practical and cost effective than oral preparations and seems to yield positive results.

14. Precursors to the important memory and cognition neurotransmitter, *acetylcholine*, may also be extremely useful to supplement with. The best sources are L-alpha glycerolphosphorylcholine (or Alpha-GPC) and dimethylaminoethinol (or DMAE). The effects are typically quite noticeable.

15. L-carnosine may be the single best protectant against glycation of brain tissue, as well as being a potent antioxidant. It has also shown significant benefits in autism. Found particularly in meat, L-carnosine tends to be deficient in vegetarian diets.

16. Glutathione precursors L-cysteine or N-acetyl cysteine (NAC), SAMe and transdermal glutathione creams (such as OxiCell and Super OxiCell by Apex Energetics) may improve levels of this critical antioxidant and anti-inflammatory substance.

17. Benfotiamine is a fat-soluble source of vitamin B1 that provides additional protection against glycation reactions, while guarding cells against the toxic effects chronic glucose exposure. Even people

with normal glucose levels encounter damaging sugar reactions over a lifetime and may benefit from some supplementation.

18. Vinpocetine is a phytonutrient that has been shown to improve memory, concentration, cognition, and cerebral circulation and has other protective effects, as well.

There are other potentially helpful supplements and techniques for improving memory, but the above covers some of the more important and better-researched approaches. Please don't feel as though you have to supplement with all this . . . but do consider following at least the basic dietary and lifestyle suggestions. They go a long way toward making a real difference!

MINERAL DEFICIENCIES AND LEARNING OR EMOTIONAL/BEHAVIORAL DISORDERS

The second-most common of all modern nutritional deficiencies includes **trace elements.** Needed in only the minutest quantities in the human body, trace elements are vital to the health of our brains and nervous systems as well as literally every other organ and function. Modern conventional agricultural practices have succeeded in depleting our soils of trace elements, and use of pesticides may block their uptake in many plants. High regional rainfall amounts can also dramatically affect soil composition and result in mineral deficient soils in many areas.

More than seventy trace elements have been identified, though comparatively few are as yet recognized as essential for health. Getting them in broad-spectrum form assures you aren't missing anything that science just hasn't gotten around to discovering the value of yet. Among the few reliable sources of broad-spectrum trace elements needed for optimal health are ocean-source seafoods, seasoning foods with unrefined, mineral-rich Celtic or Himalayan Sea salt—vastly more flavorful and healthful than conventional refined table salt—or supplementing with products like Trace Mineral Drops by Trace Minerals Research, which is relatively inexpensive and widely available.

Please avoid the use of what are called "colloidal minerals," popularized some years ago by a veterinarian named Dr. Joel Wallach.

They contain often-dangerous levels of aluminum and other toxic heavy metals and *should always be avoided* (Schauss 1997). They are also quite expensive.

The consumption of organic, biodynamically grown vegetables is also very helpful, though the mineral composition of these foods *is wholly dependent on the soil composition in which they were grown*. Minerals are, in fact, best absorbed and utilized from animal or seafood sources through ionization by hydrochloric acid and natural amino-acid chelation. *Adequate levels of hydrochloric acid, in addition to dietary fat and fat-soluble nutrients, are needed to facilitate their absorption.*

Among the macro-minerals, **zinc** deficiency is one most commonly associated with learning disabilities, ADD/HD, cognitive dysfunction, emotional lability, delinquencies and eating disorders. Zinc—also critical for immunity, healthy digestive function and found predominantly in animal source foods—is commonly deficient in those suffering from depression. Consuming significant amounts of soy, in particular, as well as large amounts of grains or legumes (due to their phytic acid) is known to cause zinc deficiencies.

Other common causes of zinc deficiency include inadequate protein intake from meat and seafood, which possess the richest natural sources, inadequate hydrochloric acid production, chronic stress, eating disorders, chronic infection and a little-known genetic metabolic condition known as pyroluria (see Appendix E). Supplementation with zinc sulfate in solution or ultra bio-available ionic zinc may be necessary, along with increased consumption of zinc-rich foods to remediate deficiency states; in tandem with other co-factors and nutrients, this can significantly improve ADD/HD symptoms. Tablets and capsules of zinc are less efficiently absorbed by those most deficient. A simple, quick and inexpensive *zinc tally* test, offered by most natural healthcare providers, can quickly, inexpensively and fairly reliably determine the presence of zinc deficiency.

Note, too, that zinc deficiency also attracts structurally similar, but highly toxic elements, such as cadmium (part of all carcinogenic processes) and mercury, which seek to replace zinc at its vacant receptor sites—a very real problem. One of the best preventatives of heavy metal toxicity is healthy mineral sufficiency!

Zinc and copper are two minerals that work together and require certain ratios to work optimally in the human body. Zinc needs to be in about an 8:1 or 12:1 ratio with copper for optimal neurological and physiological functioning. When the diet becomes deficient in zinc, or when the body loses large amounts to stress, which can *triple* its rate of excretion from the body, or in the case of diets high in phytic acid (found in soy, other legumes and grain products), the ratio moves closer to 1:1. This can result in symptoms of copper toxicity, which manifests as many of those symptoms described above (Schauss).

Zinc supplementation may be necessary in some cases where prolonged stress, deficiency or dietary inhibitors (i.e., phytic acid in grains, legumes and soy) have been prevalent for extended periods of time. Zinc monomethionine is a pill form that is preferable to many other pill forms and is commonly and inexpensively found in health food stores, though liquid ionic forms and zinc sulfate in liquid solution are far superior for absorption and bioavailability. Liquid ionic forms are best used in markedly deficient states. Safe doses for zinc are 50 mg for highly bioavailable forms and 100 mg for low bioavailable forms in average individuals. Individual needs may vary widely. Although the RDAs for this nutrient are much lower—only 15 mg for males 11+ years and 12 mg for non-pregnant or lactating females, for instance—much higher doses may be needed for a time to treat deficiency and/or specific conditions. Pyrolurics (see Appendix E) may require much higher than average levels of zinc supplementation. Average Paleolithic daily intake was probably close to about 50 mg. Note: zinc toxicity is rare in humans. Individuals on vegetarian or vegan or high soy-food diets may be especially vulnerable to zinc deficiency.

Sources in food

The best dietary sources of zinc are in foods of animal origin. Excellent sources include oysters, herring, meat, and egg yolks. Adding as little as three ounces of extra lean beef daily (again, please, organic, solely grass-fed and free range) can significantly improve zinc status. Zinc in commonly cited natural sources such as pumpkin seeds tends to have poor bioavailability, due to the presence of phytic acid and need for proper ionization (the presence of HCl)—soaking and sprouting these seeds can improve their digestibility, lower phytic acid and improve zinc availability somewhat. Note again that it is possible to induce zinc deficiency in diets rich in grains and legumes and particularly, soy. Diets high in processed foods, particularly sugar, contribute significantly to deficiency. Zinc levels are also suppressed during acute and chronic infections, pernicious anemia, alcoholism, renal disease, cardiovascular disease, some malignancies, protein calorie malnutrition and stress. Stress, alone, can more than triple one's rate of zinc excretion.

Iron and other mineral deficiencies are especially common worldwide where cereal grains make up a major portion of the diet and with vegetarian or vegan diets in general. In the past several years, researchers have found that iron deficiency is associated with often-irreversible impairment of a child's learning ability, IQ and other behavioral abnormalities. Although significant levels of non-heme iron exist in foods such as spinach and some legumes, it is poorly absorbed and utilized (roughly 1–5%). Vitamin C helps improve iron utilization from these foods somewhat. In contrast, red meat contains heme iron—the source most readily used by the human body. Iron from meat sources, particularly red meat, is not less than 20% bioavailable. The presence of heme iron in a meal also improves the absorbability from non-heme iron sources. The next best sources are poultry and fish. It is always better to replenish iron via diet rather than supplementation, as various toxicities and side effects are common with supplemental sources, particularly those such as commonly prescribed ferrous sulfate. Often simply improving hydrochloric acid production can be the single factor that makes a marked difference in mineral status.

It is important to note that excesses of iron are also a problem for some and may pose a greater threat than any other form of what is commonly termed "heavy-metal toxicity." Iron can be a powerful free-radical producer and carcinogen. Most common sources of excess iron, however, are cast-iron cookware, iron supplements, distilled alcohol, and baked goods from "enriched flours"—all of which are best avoided by everyone.

Also, however (and this is important), it is possible to have what appears to be an excessively high level of *serum* iron and even elevated ferritin, while suffering actual *intracellular* deficiencies (D. Klinghardt, MD, PhD). This is most common where chronic infections (viral, parasitic, etc.) are present and these should be ruled out. The body will use iron and copper as oxidizing agents against viruses and other microbial agents. The elevated serum levels reflect "spent" ammunition. Addressing the infection by taking high doses of vitamin C or other reducing agents to help regenerate iron and supporting immune function can turn this situation around. If excess iron toxicity is truly determined to be the case, however, the best approach is simply to get rid of your excess iron-laden blood by donating it. This is faster, cheaper and usually more effective than chelation (or some other means).

Iron deficiency symptoms can include listlessness, pallor, fatigue, apathy, impaired IQ and cognitive function, and various behavioral disorders. Although iron is commonly found in leafy greens such as spinach and some legumes, it is poorly absorbed from these sources. Red meat is the best available source, followed by poultry and fish. Deficiencies early in development can often lead to irreversible damage to

IQ, cognitive and immune function. Dietary replenishment is vastly preferable to supplemental approaches due to potential toxicities and side effects of commonly prescribed forms.

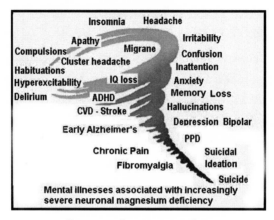

Illustration by permission from
George Eby (http//www.George-Eby-Research.com)

Magnesium insufficiency or deficiency is virtually epidemic and can be ill-afforded by a society suffering so many social, dietary and environmental stressors. Sympathetic nervous system dominance was something we were designed to be engaged in during an emergency situation . . . such as, say, being chased by a saber-toothed tiger. Today, the majority of Americans are "being chased by saber-toothed tigers" 24/7. We were designed to function in a dominantly parasympathetic state—a rarity today, indeed. Magnesium is critically important to healthy parasympathetic functioning and also to about 325+ enzymes in the body, and is readily lost with the consumption of high sugar or starch, carbohydrate foods.

Magnesium has been consistently depleted in our soils. It has been further depleted in plants by the use of potassium and phosphorus laden fertilizers which alter the plant's ability to uptake magnesium.

Water from deep wells supplies additional magnesium not found in food, but surface water, our common source of supply, lacks magnesium. Food processing removes magnesium. Broiling, steaming and boiling remove magnesium into the water or drippings. High carbohydrate and excessively high fat diets increase the need for magnesium, as do physical and mental stress. Diuretic medications and insulin further deplete total body magnesium. As we age, magnesium uptake may be impaired. Dieting reduces intake of already low levels of magnesium intake. Magnesium protects the cell from aluminum, mercury, lead, cadmium, beryllium and nickel. Evidence is mounting that low levels of magnesium contribute to the heavy metal deposition in the brain that precedes Parkinson's, multiple sclerosis and Alzheimer's. It is probable that low total body magnesium contributes to heavy metal toxicity in children and is a participant in the etiology of learning disorders (K. Sullivan).

Magnesium is one of the more overlooked and among the most depleted minerals in the modern diet. Readily depleted especially by high carbohydrate diets, deficiency can lead to high blood pressure, anxiety disorders, extremes of chronic muscle tension, impaired liver and brain function, cancer and heart disease.

Optimal dosages for adults and children may vary considerably, relative to dietary habits and whatever physical or mental demands, symptoms or issues an individual has. On average, 2.5–4.5 mg of magnesium *per pound* of ideal body weight is likely sufficient for the average healthy individual. For best absorption, smaller doses at a time (100–200 mg), two or three times a day are more optimal. Superior bioavailability may be found in forms such as ionic magnesium, magnesium glycinate or transdermal magnesium sources. Add more, if any of the symptoms on the following page apply to you, since more may temporarily be needed to replenish deficiency, or if you are particularly active or under extra stress. Cut back on supplementation if stools become too soft or loose. Ionic forms are better at avoiding this problem as they are better at absorbing intracellularly, where it is most needed, and are less likely to be readily excreted by the colon.

As it stands, most individuals can likely benefit from some magnesium supplementation . . . just remember that no nutrient functions in isolation in the body and be sure to eat foods that provide adequate minerals (including calcium) from other sources.

The following disorders are commonly associated with magnesium deficiency: (Other conditions are also associated with chronic and acute low magnesium intake and further research is continuing to confirm relationships)
- ADD/ADHD
- Alzheimer's
- Angina
- Anxiety disorders
- Arrhythmia
- Arthritis—Rheumatoid and Osteoarthritis
- Asthma
- Autism
- Auto immune disorders—all types
- Cavities
- Cerebral Palsy—in children from magnesium deficient mothers
- Chronic Fatigue Syndrome
- Congestive Heart Disease
- Constipation
- Crooked teeth—narrow jaw—in children from magnesium deficient mothers
- Depression
- Diabetes—Type I and II
- Eating disorders—Bulimia, Anorexia

- Fibromyalgia
- Gut disorders including peptic ulcer, Crohn's disease, colitis, food allergy
- Heart Disease—Arteriosclerosis, high cholesterol, high triglycerides
- Heart Disease—in infants born to magnesium deficient mothers
- High Blood Pressure
- Hypoglycemia
- Impaired athletic performance
- Infantile Seizure—in children from magnesium deficient mothers
- Insomnia
- Kidney Stones
- Lou Gehrig's Disease
- Migraines including cluster type
- Mitral Valve Prolapse
- Multiple Sclerosis
- Muscle cramps
- Muscle weakness, fatigue
- Myopia—in children from magnesium deficient mothers
- Obesity, especially obesity associated with high carbohydrate diets
- Osteoporosis—just adding magnesium reversed bone loss
- Parkinson's Disease
- PMS including menstrual pain and irregularities
- PPH (Primary Pulmonary Hypertension)
- Reynaud's
- SIDS (Sudden Infant Death Syndrome)
- Stroke
- Syndrome X—insulin resistance
- Thyroid disorders—low, high and auto-immune; low magnesium reduces T4

Unfortunately, serum blood tests are an unreliable tool for measuring magnesium levels, as they do not measure intracellular magnesium, where it is most important.

Iodine deficiency is a broadly rampant issue, and one that can impact **every** aspect of endocrine, cognitive, mood and immune function. It is easily the most under-recognized and widely impacting trace mineral deficiency problem today—an issue more recently brought to light by two independent medical doctors: Guy Abraham and David Brownstein.

Although *iodine deficiency* isn't one of the first things that comes to mind with learning disabilities, mood and cognitive dysfunction for most, this mineral is so widely deficient (and so widely misunderstood) in the American population, it likely impacts most known health problems today and cannot be ignored as a timely and critical issue.

Thyroid hormones T3 and T4 are made up of the amino acid L-tyrosine combined with either 3 or 4 molecules of iodine. Thyroid problems are growing widely and can lead to all manners of brain dysregulation, learning, memory and mood disorders. Care must be taken, however, to rule out autoimmune thyroid issues (Hashimoto's) prior to iodine supplementation. Hashimoto's cases, though particularly deficient in iodine and in need of proper supplementation, need to be clearly identified and addressed more cautiously. Iodine requires cofactors such as B-complex, C-complex, magnesium, vitamin E complex and selenium, broad spectrum trace elements (using something like Celtic sea salt) and EFA's in order to be properly absorbed into the tissues and properly utilized. It is important that tissue levels of these nutrient co-factors be healthy first. Failure to ensure this may result in uncomfortable abreactions and can even accelerate autoimmune destruction of the thyroid in susceptible individuals.

Although iodine is commonly recognized as needed for healthy thyroid functioning, many are not aware that iodine is greatly needed for the normal functioning of each and every cell, as well as normal manufacture of all hormones and functioning of the entire endocrine system (also improving the sensitivity of hormone receptors)—broadly impacting many aspects of health. Every organ and all tissues contain and *must have* iodine. The brain is no exception.

The therapeutic actions of iodine include: antibacterial, antiviral, antiparasitic, anticancer, elevates pH and can serve as a mucolytic agent (breaking up mucus in the body). Among the conditions that may be successfully improved or treated with iodine include:

- ADD
- Breast diseases
- Excess mucous production
- Fibrocystic breasts
- Headaches and migraines
- Brain fog
- Infections
- Liver diseases
- Parotid duct stones
- Prostate disorders
- Thyroid disorders
- Senility
- Goiter
- Atherosclerosis
- Dupuytren's Contracture
- Fatigue
- Hemorrhoids
- Hypertension
- Memory problems
- Keloids
- Ovarian disease
- Peyronie's
- Sebaceous cysts
- Vaginal infections
- Deafness

Apart from iodine-poor soils and reduced iodine in the food supply, one major reason for rampant iodine deficiencies involves toxic levels of other halogens in our environment, water and food supply. First on the list of offenders include bromine/bromide, included in all baked goods (as an anti-caking agent), soft drinks, sports drinks, medications, highly processed vegetable oils, many pools and spas as a disinfectant, most household items (including flame retardants in everything from carpets to electronics) and pesticides. Bromide/bromine toxicity is everywhere and affecting nearly everyone. Fluoride in municipal water supplies are also a major problem, as well as is chlorination. All these substances serve to displace iodine in the body and all its tissues, are markedly toxic, and require large doses of iodine to reverse the problem.

Taking excess amounts of iodine (or too much too quickly) can lead to uncomfortable detox reactions as these halogens are displaced. Therefore, it is important to approach iodine supplementation carefully, knowledgeably and systematically. Iodine's cofactors (previously listed) are essential to successful iodine supplementation. Good dietary sources of iodine include all seafood, kelp and other seaweeds. Iodized salt only supplies *iodide* and is not sufficient to supply all tissues with needed iodine. Only about 10% of iodine in iodized salt is actually bioavailable. Unrefined, full spectrum sea salt that is not iodized is a fairly poor source of iodine, incidentally—though very helpful with its utilization in the body. The best supplemental sources of higher potency iodine includes Prolamine iodine (protein bound and highly bioavailable—proprietary formula by Standard Process Labs), Iodoral (combines iodine and iodide, the two forms needed by the body) and Lugol's solution (mostly available by prescription). Kelp supplements may provide smaller amounts of naturally occurring iodine that are well tolerated and easily absorbed, though may be inadequate to reversing severe deficiency states or bromide/fluoride and chlorine toxicity. It can take 3–6 months of diligent iodine supplementation to reach full iodine sufficiency throughout the body (longer in some suffering more severe health challenges) and maintenance levels of iodine supplementation will likely be required long term for many.

For more information concerning the details of iodine deficiency, testing and proper supplementation protocols, look for the excellent book by Dr. David Brownstein, MD: *Iodine—Why You Need It; Why You Can't Live Without It.*

OTHER NUTRIENTS THAT MAY HELP
ALLEVIATE ADD/HD SYMPTOMS

L-tyrosine, an amino acid, together with vitamin B6, are important precursors to both norepinephrine and dopamine. These neurotransmitters are largely associated with positive mood and the brain's capacity to focus and remain alert. Depletion of these important catecholamines is commonly found in those with attentional disorders and some forms of depression. The effect of methylphenidate and other stimulants, to some degree, is to force a release of these neurotransmitters, which may ultimately be depleting (plus causing other problems). Other popular drugs such as Strattera work by inhibiting the re-uptake of these neurotransmitters. Supplementation with L-tyrosine can be a drug-free alternative to these damaging substances. Adequate B vitamins (B6, in particular) are also needed for the proper metabolic conversions. Poor protein intake, excess carbohydrate intake and poor digestion can result in amino acid deficiencies and poor neurotransmitter function. Chronic sugar or starch consumption can literally block healthy functioning of these and other neurotransmitters and also cause their depletion. Dosages used in studies ranged from up to 5,000 mg per day on an empty stomach for children, and up to 10,000 mg per day for adults. The needed dosages will vary widely and care should be given to appropriately determining individual requirements. This amino acid can also be a godsend to those addicted to stimulant drugs and may rapidly facilitate relief from these addictions, in tandem with improved diet and additional nutrients. It is important to start with the lowest dose and increase slowly every half hour on an empty stomach until the desired effect is reached to arrive at the individually-appropriate dosage. Do not over-supplement!

L-alpha-glycerylphosphorylcholine (better known as Alpha-GPC) along with **dimethylaminoethinol** (DMAE), serve as important precursors to acetylcholine—they are essential to your brain's memory and learning capacity. These substances can safely stimulate and nourish the brain in a non-addictive manner. DMAE is richly abundant in sardines, anchovies and other fish. It can also inhibit and help rid the body (skin and organs, including the brain) of lipofuscin, a pigment in the skin and brain (sometimes referred to as "age spots") normally associated with aging. Both Alpha-GPC (600–1200 mg/day) and DMAE (50–500 mg/day) can help a wide variety of cognitive and behavioral problems, as well as support healthy mood function and sleep. In one study using DMAE, hyperactive kids showed improvement in just ten weeks. In another study, children with learning disabilities did better in concentration and skill tests—all without adverse side effects such as increase in heart rate and blood pressure, agitation or unhealthy appetite suppression as with drugs. Alpha-GPC is well tolerated and widely accepted to be safe.

Acetyl L-carnitine is very structurally similar to acetylcholine. It has a variety of benefits to the brain for prevention of glycation, degenerative processes, including Alzheimer's, and improving cognitive function.

L-tryptophan or 5-HTP can be helpful in cases of hyperactivity. For a young child, 25 mg of 5-HTP may be a good starting dose, to be incrementally increased, as needed, or 250 mg of L-tryptophan on an empty stomach. (Not both.) If sleep is also an issue, L-tryptophan may be the better choice. Sugar consumption can disrupt the therapeutic effect.

Vinpocetine (10–20 mg, 3 or 4 times a day), a supplemental phytonutrient, can significantly improve cerebral circulation and cognitive functioning. It has effects on brain blood vessels, brain blood flow, and even brain cells themselves. Many report improved concentration ability. Vinpocetine can be of value in enhancing the delivery of oxygen and nutrients to the brain, as well as in possibly preventing the damage that occurs if nutrient delivery is impaired. According to some research, it may also help to prevent the neurotoxic effects implicated in Alzheimer's disease. It also has antioxidant properties and has been shown to improve memory.

RELIEF FROM ANXIETY AND DEPRESSION IN OUR UNCERTAIN WORLD

Anxiety and depression are easily the most prevalent psychological disorders today and commonly co-exist together in those who are afflicted. They are epidemic. Major depression, alone, is expected to be the second leading cause of disability by 2020 *worldwide*—second only to ischemic heart disease (Institute of Functional Medicine). In the United States, a quarter of the population is at risk for major depression.

I personally suffered intractable depression and chronic dysthymia for thirty-five or more years before I discovered neurofeedback. Along with depression, I also suffered anxiety and panic attacks that altogether defined my entire existence for far too long. The symptoms robbed me of my full experience of life and continually weighed like a dark cloud over every pursuit. I used to liken it to swimming with ankle weights on—periodically getting up a head of steam and fighting my way to the surface into the fresh air and sunlight, where I could drink in the air and make some headway in my life—only to eventually be weighted back down into the black, smothering depths of despair and futility. As time went on, these bouts became more frequent, insidious, prolonged and severe. It almost came to a point where I could not see the point in fighting my way back to the surface any longer. In some ways, I really just didn't want to be here anymore.

Today, it's hard to imagine having ever been there. For the last twelve years or more, now, this has been a total non-issue for me. I can remember well what it was like, and feel deep empathy for others similarly suffering. Let's just say "I get it."

A common misconception about depression is that it is somehow a "lazy" person's disorder and that all anyone has to do is simply pull themselves up by their own bootstraps and "get it together." Depression is in actuality a state of "chronic efforting." It's a state of spinning one's wheels in the freshly fallen snow (I'm originally from Minnesota; snow analogies work for me.) Your wheels spin and spin until smoke starts coming from the transmission. Eventually you run out of gas and wear down the engine. For too many, the solution is simply to get more gas . . . when what you really need is to stop, let the tires cool, then ease gently out of the ditch. (There's your crash course in Minnesota winter driving, 101.)

For the majority of those I see, depression is really a state of "anxiety to exhaustion." It is a state of learned helplessness.

Although the answer for me was ultimately neurofeedback—for which I will be eternally grateful and devoted—knowing what I know today about diet would, I believe, have made a major difference in that equation for me, much sooner.

Make no mistake: insulin and leptin are major players in this equation. Both hormones, when elevated, stimulate sympathetic over-arousal and can easily provoke agitative and exhausting anxiety states. Advanced glycation processes additionally degenerate the brain, damaging the brain's natural inhibitory capacity and sending it into chronic sympathetic overdrive. Deficiencies of amino acids (due to digestive problems or protein poor diets), iodine, zinc, magnesium, B-complex, EFA's and others fuel the problem. Add this to acute—or even average—life stressors and the effect can be quite punctuated, if not intolerable. Fluctuations in blood sugar further destabilize the system and mood, adding to cortisol problems. Elevated stress hormones, as a result of the insulin and leptin surges, stimulate even more insulin, which, in turn, cause the kidneys to dump magnesium which is necessary for relaxed, parasympathetic functioning.

Chronic adrenal dysregulation in women can lead to deficiencies of estrogen at menopause. This diminished estrogen in women lowers serotonin receptor activity, leading to commonly reported depression issues in post-menopausal women. Abnormally diminished estrogen also results in cerebral inflammation and subsequent brain degeneration. In men, dysglycemia and concomitant adrenal dysregulation can cause similar depression in testosterone levels, which, in turn, depresses dopamine function.

Furthermore (as you may recall), our rate of zinc excretion goes up several-fold under stress, and our requirement for B vitamins—essential for healthy nervous system functioning—rises sharply and is depleted rapidly by stress and chronic carbohydrate consumption. Sympathetic over-arousal also shuts down digestion and hydrochloric acid production (further compromised by dietary carbohydrates), additionally blocking the absorption of important minerals and preventing the proper digestion of protein into amino acids needed for neurotransmitter production. We rapidly lose electrolytes under stress and our body's bioelectrical system suffers, neurological timing mechanisms suffer, and the system struggles for equilibrium. EFAs get used up rapidly battling elevations in inflammatory cytokines induced by leptin surges, which rapidly destroy mitochondria, energy levels and our need for omega-3s climbs.

We're drained of our reserves. The brain suffers. Energy plummets.

We see the entire world around us through this chaotic biochemical lens. Life looks bleak, if not overwhelming. For some, this is entirely identifiable as a state of chronic anxiety. For others, it spirals and descends into depression or some combined state of misery.

Are you seeing the common thread here?

Food sensitivities, EMF pollution and everyday stressors add another layer to the draining mix. Adrenals move progressively toward exhaustion; the thyroid suffers. One seeks alcohol or carbohydrate-rich snacks to help stimulate struggling serotonin levels, while actually further depleting them, and/or dissociating you from everyday reality. And so, the cycle self-perpetuates.

Life sucks.

Author, scholar, CIA analyst and professor emeritus, Chalmers Ashby Johnson said about the U.S. military-industrial complex, "I guarantee you when war becomes profitable; you are going to see more of it." In exactly the same manner, as physical and mental illness has become extremely profitable, we are seeing and will continue to see more of it. In 1985, the total annual sales for all anti-depressants in the United States was approximately $240 million; today it is in excess of $12 *billion*. Between 1987 and 1997, the percentage of Americans in outpatient treatment for depression more than tripled. Of those in treatment, the percentage of prescribed medication nearly doubled.

Depression is not a Prozac deficiency. Anxiety is not a deficiency of any pharmaceutical anxielytic agent.

Personal issues certainly cloud the equation, but psychotherapy is ill-suited to get at the physiological underpinnings that are "depression" or "anxiety." Both disorders are commonly the product of a vicious cycle that becomes self-perpetuating and colors the lens through which life is experienced. It is a substantially tainted lens.

Improved diet, digestion and nutrient repletion is everything to these pop-ulations.

Neurofeedback can sometimes dramatically help restore healthy timing and better self-regulation . . . but it is diet that ultimately corrects the underlying biochemistry. The brain simply needs certain raw materials to work with; it also needs to be able to get other things which simply don't belong there out of the way.

Although all this might sound very complex—but the basic foundational formula and dietary approach (presented all along in this book) is actually quite simple. *Most* supplements are optional.

NUTRIENTS TO SUPPORT DEPRESSION AND ANXIETY

► Very low carbohydrate, moderate protein and sufficient fat intake as needed to satisfy appetite, including supplementation with omega-3s and GLA (i.e., black currant seed oil)

► Adequate hydration

► B-complex supplementation

► Trace Mineral Drops or use of full-spectrum (i.e., Celtic or Himalayan) sea salt

► Magnesium (600–800mg/day)—Magnesium glycinate is a highly bioavailable form. Liquid ionic forms may be better utilized by those with impaired digestion and may also reach intracellular levels more effectively. Liquid ionic magnesium may also be effective at much smaller doses

► Zinc (either ionic form or amino acid chelated)

► L-tryptophan (comes in 500 mg caps)—May be useful for both anxiety and depression symptoms and is a direct precursor to serotonin. A widely available metabolite, 5-hydroxytryptophan (5-HTP), may also be helpful but may additionally raise cortisol levels (which may not be desirable for some, especially if sleep is an issue). Start with one capsule of L-tryptophan on an empty stomach, notice how you are feeling, if no enhanced sense of well being after 20–30 minutes, take another capsule . . . and so on. When a positive shift is experienced, that is your dose. Do not take, if you are also taking antidepressants, unless under careful qualified medical supervision

▸ For anxiety coupled with mind racing and physical tension, the amino acid, Theanine can be wonderful. Start with a low dose (on an empty stomach) and work up in dosage the same way as L-tryptophan. Take only what is needed to achieve better relaxation. (200–400 mg/day). Found in green and black tea, it can serve as a precursor to the primary inhibitory or calming neurotransmitter, gamma-aminobutyric acid (GABA), which may also be used supplementally. Theanine also has known positive effects on serotonin and dopamine levels. Smaller doses may be mildly stimulating, while larger doses tend to be quite calming. It has also been shown to lower high blood pressure. It readily crosses the blood-brain barrier and may be significantly neuroprotective, especially with impaired cerebral circulation

▸ Gamma-aminobutyric acid (GABA)—both an amino acid and an inhibitory (calming) neurotransmitter GABA may be successfully used for issues concerning anxiety, racing thoughts and physical tension. Though oral GABA cannot normally cross the healthy, intact blood-brain barrier, wide ranging benefit is often reported with supplementation.

▸ Taurine—another amino acid very useful for anxiety-related issues and instabilities. Taurine is the end-product of sulfur metabolism and an antioxidant. It is a constituent of healthy bile and can help support biliary function as well. Taurine has its highest concentrations in electrically conductive tissue such as the brain, the heart and the nervous system. It greatly helps curb excitatory activity and nervousness without being sedating. Also, high concentrations of taurine occur naturally in the retina of the eye. There is no known toxicity. Taurine comes in 500 mg capsules and can be taken in a similar fashion as the other aminos. Usually 1,000–2,000 mg does the trick, but some need more or less. Very high doses in excess of 5,000 mg can result in a diuretic effect (but one that spares electrolytes). Taurine tends to be very safe and well tolerated by most.

▸ L-tyrosine is a precursor to norepinephrine and dopamine, two neurotransmitters commonly associated with some forms of depression. L-tyrosine comes in 500 mg capsules and may be taken the same way as other aminos. It has a stimulant effect and may be inappropriate for those in active or acute stress response (it may worsen or cause agitation). Also, don't use L-tyrosine if you have malignant melanoma (it is a precursor to melanin). Don't use it if anxiety is a significant part of the problem for you

▸ DL-phenylalanine (DLPA)—Yet another amino acid precursor to both L-tyrosine and norepinephrine and dopamine, as well as beta-endorphins. Same restrictions apply as to L-tyrosine. The D-fraction may be especially useful where there is pain or tendency toward "addiction to pleasure-seeking stimuli," as it helps specifically enhance the function of endorphins

▸ Light Boxes (light, after all, is decidedly a nutrient!)—Where Seasonal Affective Disorder issues are present, these light boxes, which emit up to 10,000 LUX may be extremely useful and transformative of mood and circadian rhythms. Use for 15–30 minutes in the morning to shut down undesirable chronic inappropriate melatonin production. This may help lessen fatigue or depression during the day, and significantly enhance serotonin production. If staying asleep at night is a significant problem, using the light box later in the afternoon or early evening (at least two hours before bedtime) can improve sleep quality, too. Spending some time outdoors at around noontime daily (an hour, or so if possible) is another natural means of getting adequate "light nutrition." Avoid sunscreens or even sunglasses if possible. Being in the shade is okay

▸ Vitamin D deficiency has also been identified as deficient in those with Seasonal Affective Disorder, as well as other forms of mood dysregulation and supplementation should be considered. Read the chapter earlier in this book on Vitamin D for supplementation and dosage guidelines.

Note:

▸ Competition with each other for metabolic transport sites across the blood-brain barrier tends to make supplementation of amino acids most effective when specifically desired amino acids are taken in isolation from one another, on an empty stomach, and in the absence of dietary protein.

▸ Transport of amino acids across the blood-brain barrier are blocked by elevated glucose.

▸ Most amino acids require the presence of co-factors and accessory nutrients to make proper conversions into neurotransmitters. B6 (also known as Pyridoxal-5-phosphate, or P-5-P) is most often needed and is depleted by all antidepressant medications. Other commonly need-ed nutrients for proper neurotransmitter conversions include iron for both serotonin and dopamine, and folic acid, which is commonly deficient. Always be sure you are supplementing with B-complex at mealtime and that you are not anemic.

▸ Symptoms experienced are probably the best indicator of which amino acid is likely to work best for you. Although urinary neu-rotransmitter testing has gained some popularity, the approach is deeply flawed, inaccurate and very expensive. It is far better to rely on symptoms as the most accurate available indicator of neurotransmit-ter deficiency.

▸ Amino acids tend to be self-weaning over time and are far safer and faster acting than nearly all prescribed medications used to treat the same symptoms. In most cases, the effects may be readily experienced within minutes to hours, rather than days or weeks. Long term, a bet-ter diet is likely to be your best insurance for sustained mental health.

The following are common symptoms associated with various neu-rotransmitter deficiencies and the amino acids most effective in re-plenishing your brain's supply.

Serotonin deficiency symptoms (may respond to L-tryptophan or 5-HTP):

- Depressed
- Worried and anxious
- Negative thinking
- Seasonal Affective Disorder (SAD) symptoms
- Anger or Aggressiveness
- Poor sleep
- Shy or fearful
- Loss of pleasure in things you used to enjoy
- Crave carbohydrates

Note: Iron is needed for the conversion of L-tryptophan to sero-tonin. Anemia may make this conversion very difficult in some. It is important to rule this out.

Dopamine deficiency symptoms (may respond to L-tyrosine or L-phenylalanine):

- Depression
- Lacking physical or mental energy
- Low libido
- Poor self-esteem
- Poor motivation or enthusiasm
- Distractible
- Short fuse
- Crave stimulants and carbohydrates

Note: Iron or folic acid is needed for the conversion of L-tyrosine to L-Dopa. Anemia may make this conversion very difficult in some. It is important to rule this out.

GABA deficiency symptoms (may respond to GABA, Theanine and/or Taurine):

- Racing thoughts
- Inability to relax or "loosen up"
- Poor sleep
- Feeling anxious or panicky for no reason
- Feelings of impending doom
- Crave alcohol, food, nicotine or drugs to "calm down"

Endorphin deficiency symptoms (may respond to DL-Phenylalanine or particularly D-Phenylalanine):

- Extra-sensitive to emotional or physical pain
- Cry or tear-up too easily
- Avoid painful issues
- Chronic physical or emotional pain issues
- Crave "comfort foods" or "numbing" indulgences

Precautions

Avoid taking the following amino acids

- L-TYROSINE or L-/DL-PHENYLALANINE: *if* you are prone to migraines, on antidepressants, have high blood pressure, or suffer from bipolar/manic depression
- L-GLUTAMINE/L-TRYPTOPHAN, 5-HTP: *if* you have a carcinoid tumor
- GABA/TAURINE: *if* you have very low blood pressure

SO HOW DOES EXERCISE
FIT INTO THIS EQUATION?

Studies show that simply walking three times a week in older adults can improve measurements of focus and attention. Some research even indicates that gray matter volume within several brain regions, including the frontal and temporal cortex, is larger in people (women, in particular) who regularly exert themselves aerobically. Exercise has been shown to have an equal, if not superior effect on mood to SSRI medications.

Animal studies show that exercise increases the expression of the neurotransmitter receptors involved in "brain plasticity" (the ability of the brain to function more flexibly) and learning, and enables animals' brains to generate new neurons. Clearly, exercise is a decidedly helpful thing, and can also improve oxygenation and circulation to all tissues—including the brain.

Emotion is created by motion
—TONY ROBBINS

By moving our bodies, we engage a greater and more flexible capacity for emotion. More than 100 studies done regarding the impact of exercise on anxiety and depression have shown a consistent and significantly positive benefit, roughly equal to most traditional therapies. In addition, other variables positively affected by exercise include generally improved mood, enhanced self-esteem, improved ability to recover from psychosocial stressors and more restful sleep. Recent studies have found that exercise boosts activity in the brain's frontal lobes and the hippocampus. Animal studies have found that exercise effectively increases levels of serotonin, dopamine and norepinephrine—all associated with enhanced mood function.

Exercise has also been found to increase levels of Brain-Derived Neurotrophic Factor (BDNF), which is thought to help improve mood and also help brain cells survive longer. This, in turn, points to the role of exercise in additionally benefiting and/or helping prevent dementia—it's about a lot more than just enhanced endorphin production. Everyone should find a way to engage in something physical and something they enjoy.

In the largely sedentary society in which we live, we need to remember to get outdoors into the fresh air and sunshine, and move our bodies in ways it was designed to move. Adding oxygen and circulation to the equation can only add positive benefit in the quest for mental health.

WHAT ABOUT FOOD ALLERGIES AND SENSITIVITIES?

Food allergies and sensitivities are an extensive and complex subject and an extremely common problem among those with learning disabilities and other behavioral, physiological, emotional and neurological problems. Frequently, symptoms can easily resemble nutrient deficiencies and heavy metal toxicities as well as traumatically generated psychological disorders. Doris J. Rapp, MD, lists the following nervous system symptoms as possible signs of food allergies or sensitivities:

- Hyperactive, wild, unrestrained
- Talkative (explosive, stuttering, constant)
- Inattentive, disruptive, impulsive
- Short attention span
- Restless legs, finger tapping
- Clumsiness, in coordination, tremor
- Insomnia, nightmares
- Nervous, irritable, upset, short-tempered
- High strung, excitable, agitated
- Moody, tired, weak, weary, exhausted, listless, depressed
- Easily moved to tears, easily hurt
- Highly sensitive to odor, light, sound, pain and cold

Other medical symptoms as related to food allergies or sensitivities:
- Nose: year-round stuffiness, watery nose, sneezing, nose rubbing

- Aches: head, back, neck, muscles or joints—e.g., "growing pains"—or aches unrelated to exercise
- Belly problems: bellyaches, nausea, upset stomach, bloating, bad breath, gassy stomach, belching
- Bladder problems: wetting pants in daytime or in bed, need to rush to urinate, burning or pain with urination
- Face: pale, dark eye circles, puffiness below eyes
- Glands: swelling of lymph nodes of neck
- Ear Problems: repeated formation of fluid behind eardrums, ringing ears, dizziness
- Excessive perspiration
- Low-grade fever

Elimination diets are the most inexpensive and accurate method to determine whether food allergies or sensitivities are to blame for such symptoms but require patience and disciplined effort. By eliminating suspected culprits—the most common are grains, soy, corn, peanuts, chicken eggs and dairy—for a period of time (no less than one week—two weeks is better). Then, in reintroducing each of these, one at a time every 72 hours, a determination can usually be made. The effects become obvious either immediately or within that 72 hours.

Often times the food an individual craves most is to blame and can be a strong hint indicating where to start. Some health professionals offer other varying forms of testing in this area, though most testing is expensive and/or varies somewhat in accuracy.

A highly accredited company called EnteroLab (www.enterolab. com) has perhaps the single best and most accurate available means of diagnosing sensitivities to the most common food substances. They use a proprietary stool antigen test. Anyone may order a test kit by contacting them, without a prescription. The prevalence of gluten and casein sensitivities alone make this testing indispensable for almost everyone, particularly where unexplained health issues of any kind are present. The Web site is also an invaluable source of accurate information. Insurance reimbursement with EnteroLab may be possible.

Wherever food allergies or sensitivities are a problem, digestion can be a core cause (review chapter on digestion). Essentially, the problem begins when undigested food particles pass inappropriately through a compromised intestinal wall (via leaky gut syndrome) and become antigens—targets for your immune system. With a healthy gut this should not happen. Re-establishing gut and digestive health and integrity is critical for long-term recovery.

> **Digestive issues are critical to consider where learning, attentional, autoimmune, cognitive or emotional/behavioral problems exist. Restoring normal digestion and healthy gastrointestinal flora should be among the first steps taken toward improving these conditions.**

Some food allergies and sensitivities may both be cyclic in nature and respond to several months' abstinence—after which one may reincorporate certain offending foods in a limited way. Other sensitivities (commonly gluten and casein) may require permanent and complete abstinence. Where autoimmune conditions and autism (which may be categorized as an autoimmune brain disorder) are concerned, food sensitivities—particularly gluten and casein—should be assumed, and these foods completely eliminated. Results of successful, long term elimination for many can be dramatic.

Exploring the possibility of food sensitivities or allergies is a potentially very worthwhile consideration when dealing with a seemingly inexplicable array of symptoms. Two very informative books on the subject include *Allergies and the Hyperactive Child* by Doris J. Rapp, MD and *Is This Your Child?* by Doris J. Rapp, MD. Another more

recently published superb book on this subject that is highly recommended is *Gut and Psychology Syndrome: Natural Treatment for
Autism, Dyspraxia, Dyslexia, ADD/ADHD, Depression and Schizo-
phenia* by Natasha Campbell-McBride, MD, MMedSci (neurology),
MMedSci (nutrition). The Gluten-free/casein-free Web site also contains quite a bit of information: www.gfcfdiet.com.

Additional issues to consider, where one finds learning disabilities,
ADD/HD, delinquent or unexplained violent behavior, mood swings
and seeming psychiatric disorders, include heavy metal toxicity and
food additive or salicylate reactions. Visual and/or auditory processing deficits can also manifest in many learning disabilities. Seek appropriate professional assistance for diagnosis and treatment.

THE IMPACT OF MODERN DIETARY AND ENVIRONMENTAL STRESS ON THE BRAIN

This subject could be a whole book, unto itself. Our primal mind literally has no defense against the stressful world it now faces, and we are paying a terrifying price for it. We are inundated from all sides by a chemical (pollutant, excitotoxin), societal, media and electro-magnetic (EMF) onslaught—as well as our dietary self-induced tidal waves of insulin and leptin—relentlessly generating damaging excitatory activity in our brains. It is unprecedented in our history. The toll this takes is insidious as well as profound, and must be appreciated if steps are to be taken to mitigate its effects.

The richest repository of cortisol receptors in the brain lies in the hippocampus, which exists as part of our temporal lobes (right above both ears). The hippocampus is a part of our brain's limbic system. It serves a role in the formation of new memories and the retrieval of older memories, as well as spatial navigation and affect (emotion) regulation. It is typically the first area of the brain affected in Alzheimer's disease and other forms of degeneration. The hippocampus is the part of our brain most responsible for mitigating stress response, as evidenced by the preponderance of cortisol (our major stress hormone) receptors—present here more than in any other area of the brain.

Unfortunately, we were never designed to be bombarded with stress 24/7; this delicate and sensitive part of the brain can become significantly damaged from excess and chronic exposure to stress hormones and excitatory activity . Its cells can literally wither, degenerate over time and die-off, creating impaired memory function and even psychological disturbances ranging from anxiety to paranoia and emotional instability. Modern imaging studies increasingly show a common trend in the general population toward the obvious signs of shrinkage, and "Swiss cheese"-looking temporal lobe degeneration in many. This is now being referred to clinically as a "normal variant of aging" by radiologists. The fact that it is so very common, however, hardly makes it "normal."

This dangerous trend underscores the need for stress reduction as a mandatory practice for everyone. Neurofeedback can be an especially powerful mitigator of chronic stress, as well as teaching vastly improved self-regulation of excitatory neurological activity. In my neurofeedback practice, every client gets some form of temporal lobe training to help calm the damaging excitatory activity there that is typical for most. Neurofeedback often dramatically improves self-regulation of stress-related circuitry. Other methods of biofeedback may also be extremely useful for stress-reduction, including especially heart-rate variability (HRV) training (www.HeartMath.com) and capnotherapy, or "breath training" (http://www.betterphysiology.com/).

This bombardment of stress also underscores the need for lowered insulin levels, anti-glycating nutrients (L-carnosine, acetyl L carnitine, fat soluble B1, benfotiamine and fat soluble B6, pyradoxamine), as well as supplemental adaptogens (stress-mitigating herbs) such as eleuthero-ginseng, ashwagandha, maca, holy basil, rhodiola, schisandra and others—and regenerating/cortisol-attenuating and other protective nutrient substances, such as (particularly) phosphatidyl serine, B12 (and other methyl donors), and CoQ10.

Most of all, the impact of stress on the vulnerable brain may be the best argument yet for minimizing the excitatory effects of excess insulin and leptin, and the oxidizing and glycating effects of glucose.

Another point worthy of ample consideration is the impact of chronic excitatory activity on our frontal lobes—our "executive brain." This is the part of the brain that, in many ways, makes us most "human." It controls many aspects of short-term memory, inhibitory activity, consequential thinking, focus, planning and affect regulation or emotion. This part of the brain is usually not fully developed until we are in our early twenties—as reflected in the sometimes erratic and irresponsible tendencies of juveniles. As mature adults, however, this part of our brain allows us to better consider our environment, effectively use our short-term memory, properly focus, process our thoughts, plan our actions thoughtfully and control erratic impulses.

What we are really talking about when we talk about "over-arousal," "excess sympathetic nervous system activity," or "excitatory activity," is basically a state of "fight or flight." As mentioned before, this part of our nervous systems was designed to kick-in only under threatening extremes, such as being chased by a saber-toothed tiger. We live in a society today where many of us are being "chased by saber-toothed tigers" 24/7. Many people have nervous systems that function habitually in this way. They often end up seeking neurofeedback (if they're lucky), medications or other drugs and alcohol to manage this constant hellish "hijacking" of their brains. Many constantly feel like prisoners of their own nervous systems.

What is the impact—not only on us, individually, but on our society as a whole—when everyone functions in this way?

In a state of "fight or flight," our frontal lobes, our executive functioning, as described above . . . and even our "human-ness" basically shuts down. We become either purely instinctive animals or machine-like. Our judgment suffers. We lack any meaningful consideration of future or past. We're stuck in "survival mode" only. We *react,* as opposed to *respond,* to the world around us, and we become impulsive, unfocused and fail to adequately contemplate the consequences of our actions. It's adolescence run amok. It's a recipe for societal degeneration and chaos . . . and all this has become a mainstream hallmark of the society in which we live.

The ravages of insulin, leptin, excitotoxins and chronic EMF exposure are deteriorating more than just our minds . . .

They are deteriorating our entire society.

Summing it up

Suffice it to say that consuming a diet closely paralleling that of our ancient human ancestors is the best general insurance we have to avoid dietary deficiency, mental illness and cognitive decline. Although not perfect and incomplete, it is also our best available blueprint for the optimal functioning of our minds, emotions, immune systems and overall physiology.

Optimizing nutrient ratios by the elimination of simple sugars and starches, and moderating protein intake and adequate intake of healthy fat to satisfy appetite can additionally serve to greatly enhance both quantity and quality of life and takes these foundational "Paleolithic principles" to a whole new level.

From a physiological perspective, what we eat ultimately accounts for easily 70% of our health and longevity. The very foods we eat are responsible for controlling, modifying and regulating our genetic expression. This is huge. Supplementation with commonly deficient nutrients, antioxidants and anti-glycating nutrients and engaging in regular exercise can further benefit the equation and slow degenerative mental, physical and emotional decline.

Attitude, beliefs, habitual emotions and stress are less quantifiable but also enormously important. Still, the better we eat, the better the raw materials with which to manufacture "the molecules of emotion"—to borrow from Candice Pert—hormones, neurotransmitters and prostaglandins.

> Emotions, after all, are little more than biochemical "storms" in the body/mind. A healthy diet invariably makes for a better "forecast."

Emotions are not, in essence, the result of what happens to you . . . but rather, *how you respond* to what happens to you. A balanced biochemistry allows us to respond, rather than react to the world around us.

The quality this lends our experience of life cannot be underestimated.

It's not really about "living forever." It's about being healthy enough to live fully, live healthfully and live happily. Of course, the longer we are able to do this, the better.

Isn't that really the point of it all—quality of life?

We don't beat the Reaper by living longer. We beat the Reaper by living well . . . and living fully.
—RANDY PAUSCH, PHD, Professor at Carnegie-Mellon University— died July 25th, 2008, at age 47 of pancreatic cancer

PART THREE:
PARADISE LOST

*Cancer, like insanity seems to increase with
the progress of civilization.*
—STANISLAS TANCHOU, FRENCH PHYSICIAN,
MID-NINETEENTH CENTURY

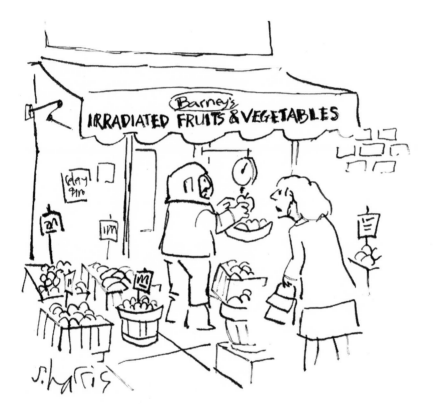

We live in uniquely perilous times. Our ancestors never would have imagined a world where meals came in cardboard boxes, or meat sources were comprised of animals filled with dangerous chemicals, hormones and fed unnatural foods, forced to live in torturous and unnatural environments. They couldn't conceive of anything such as air and water pollution, heavy metal contamination (much of this was not an issue prior to mining), electromagnetic frequency pollution (EMFs), 24-hour daylight (in the form of electricity), 10-hour work days, the stress of daily rush-hour traffic, pesticides on plant-foods, or depleted nutrients in the soils where plant foods grow. How could they have even begun to fathom "Genetically Modified Organisms" (GMOs), corrupt pharmaceutical interests, or corporate controlled FDA politics?

For us today, the challenges are much different than what we faced in our day-to-day primitive past. I personally would almost rather deal with being chased by a saber-toothed tiger or a charging cantankerous wooly mammoth then deal with the corruptive influence of the FDA, multi-national corporations, or massively contaminated food, water and air supplies.

Our environment—food, water and air supply—has decidedly, even radically, changed, even where our physiology has not. This is not a happy conundrum. How do we manage in the face of all this? How do we adapt, much less survive, at all?

Then again, some things, nowadays, are to our advantage. We no longer suffer the same sort of food shortages our ancestors did, we're less vulnerable to fearsome predators (of the four-legged variety), and we have the field of modern scientific research to occasionally give us an edge over nature, by helping to reveal her secrets. These advantages unfortunately, are mostly outweighed by the sheer burdensome toxicity and unscrupulous and deteriorating extremes of our modern society.

It's clear our challenges have changed, and once again our species is being forced to adapt—this time to a radically accelerated state of cataclysmic change to our environment on nearly all levels. The cartoon at the beginning of this chapter seems amusing. However, as of

August 21, 2008, the FDA approved the irradiation of all commercially sold spinach and lettuce—without any consumer labeling whatsoever. This effectively destroys all phytonutrients and many heat-labile vitamins (Bs and C) entirely.

Microwaving alone, for instance, destroys 98% of all phytonutrients and vitamins in vegetables and other foods. There may no longer be any cancer-preventative effect from cruciferous vegetables or any other plant food, if irradiation of all fruits and vegetables is allowed or otherwise mandated. What's next? How can we possibly survive the accelerating destruction of our food supply and environment? And where are these "modern challenges" leading us? These are among the most important questions addressed in this book, and in our time.

EMF Pollution . . . the New Tobacco?

EMF Pollution may be the most significant form of pollution human activity has produced in this century, all the more dangerous because it is invisible and insensible.
—ANDREW WEIL, MD

EMF pollution affects us all in insidious ways, we've barely begun to recognize. EMF pollution is known to generate and/or exacerbate damaging (even mutating) excitatory activity in the brain and may well be the single greatest influence on the exponential increase in anxiety-related disorders, autism, as well as brain cancers.

As a clinical Neurofeedback Specialist, I have personally observed a radical trend over the last ten years toward "high-arousal" disorders and have witnessed a nearly exponentially disproportionate shift toward the over-arousal spectrum of neurological dysregulation. Doing the work that I do has put me in the unique position of making these observations, where they may have been less noticeable for many.

After exploring the potential reasons for this, I have concluded that EMF pollution and the exponential increase in cellular towers over just the last ten years, cordless phones, wi-fi technology and home electronics best accounts for this overwhelming, rather sudden and disturbing shift.

A cursory search using the web site: www.antennasearch.com revealed no less than 67 cell towers within less than four miles of my own home. They are everywhere . . . and multiplying. The telecom industry even offers school districts money in exchange for permission to build these damaging radio wave producing behemoths on school premises, strongly exposing children's vulnerable, developing brains to certain known and unknown EMF dangers.

As with the consequences of the use of tobacco, the consequences of EMF exposure are carefully concealed by the industries that generate it and, as such, may not be fully understood and appreciated for many years (if ever) . . . by which time it may be too late. Unlike cigarettes or second-hand smoke, there is literally no escape from EMF—it surrounds and penetrates us all. The best we can do is try to minimize its impact by taking the following precautions and support our innate resilience to stress and overall health.

Minimize EMF influence by unplugging electrical appliances when not in use, especially in the room where you sleep. Minimize the use of cell phones and always use their speaker-phone option. Avoid Bluetooth and all but EMF-protective (i.e., "blue tube"—*not* "Bluetooth") headsets. Keep away from "wireless routers" and high-tension power lines. Minimize or eliminate the use of cordless phones at home and at the office. (Yes, even cordless phones are bad . . . and likely even worse than cell phones!).

It's time to start taking the EMF threat seriously and take whatever steps we can to protect from and/or compensate for its insidious biological effects.

WHAT GENERATION OF
POTTENGER'S CAT ARE YOU?

Years ago, in the 1930s, a scientist and doctor by the name of Francis Pottenger initiated a series of now famous feeding experiments with cats that spanned over ten years and several feline generations. His findings transformed for many the view of the role that diet plays in health and reproduction.

Certain groups of these cats were fed quality, fresh, un-denatured food and others varying degrees of denatured or processed food, then the effects were observed over several generations. The results were not so startling with the inferior diets for the first generation animals, but markedly and progressively so in subsequent generations. The dramatic degeneration of the genetic expression in these animals over generations casts a clear mirror image of our current health and social challenges as humans in modern society. Subsequent generations of cats fed processed and denatured diets showed increasing levels of structural deformity, birth defects, stress-driven behaviors, vulnerability to illness, allergies, reduced learning ability, and, finally, major reproductive problems. When he attempted to reverse the effects in the genetically weakened and vulnerable second-generation animals with greatly improved diet, he found it took fully four generations for the cats to return to normal.

The reflection the work of Francis Pottenger casts on the health issues and dietary habits of modern day society are glaring and inescapable.

The time has come for us to decide just what level of health we choose to have for ourselves and our children. *The choice is truly ours.* A true state of health cannot be achieved by simply "managing" a disease process with either supplements or pharmaceuticals. Supplements can, at least, help—but, by definition, they are S-U-P-P-L-E-M-E-N-T-S to a more fundamentally essential healthy approach to diet. Also, we must somehow compensate for what we are being bombarded by from all sides.

Overwhelming modern day circumstances have essentially eliminated our margin for error. The time for innocent indulgence has passed. We may no longer exercise the hubris of pretending we can get away with eating whatever we want, even "in moderation" and somehow avoid unforgiving consequences, simply because we are in denial of them. The consequences of ignorance, for many, will be beyond help. We are too many unhealthy generations of "Pottenger's cats" into the Industrial Revolution and the ravages of a deteriorating food supply and too genetically compromised by all this to indulge in a dietary approach merely dictated by one's superficial tastes (i.e., "comfort" or junk food) or wishful ideals (i.e., vegetarianism/veganism). Many no longer know the same resilience of even a generation ago.

With respect to the modern health care crisis we—*as individuals*— need to take adult responsibility for our own short sightedness and self-indulgent practices. We basically need to grow up. No one else will ever fix this for us.

There is a real danger in this time of growing economic fear to shortchange the quality of the food we eat by leaning on cheap processed and/or starch-based foods as a means of saving money. It is utterly critical we do not allow ourselves to be seduced by this thinking. Where it makes obvious sense to save money on unnecessary luxuries at such an uncertain time, a healthy, quality diet and necessary supplementation should never be viewed as any sort of "luxury"— ESPECIALLY now. If you can't afford to get sick, then you can't afford not to take your preventative health care seriously. More than ever everyone needs to be encouraged to prioritize quality food and needed supplementation as the ultimate answer to the costly health care crisis. Preventative medicine is **pennies on the dollar** as compared to the cost (on all too many levels) of falling prey to the so-called "health care system."

> Our future as a species essentially lies in our past. Adopting a dietary approach that is consistent with our foundational primitive physiological requirements is the first critical step in restoring our health. It may well be the underlying key to our very survival.

How do we possibly adapt to what we face?

I again hypothesize we are now living in a world and in a time where there is no longer any room for error with respect to what we must do to maintain our health and survival. The work of Dr. Francis Pottenger has shown us that progressive generations of poor dietary habits result in an increasingly more vulnerable progeny . . . and that each subsequent generation of unhealthy dietary habits results in impaired resistance to disease, increasingly poor health and vitality, impaired mental and cognitive health and impaired capacity to reproduce. It is all part of what we are seeing in our epidemic levels of poor health and of overwhelming rates of autism, violence, attentional disorders, childhood (and adult) behavioral problems, mental illness, fertility issues and birth defects.

We are a few generations of "Pottenger's cats," as humans, past the dawn of the Industrial Revolution and the ever-tightening tendrils of the unscrupulous, greed-driven Food Industry it spawned. We, as a species, have never been more vulnerable. The increasingly widespread consumption of processed and fast foods today and its effects are glaringly (if not disturbingly) clear. Add this to an increasingly contaminated environment, corrupt and broken healthcare system and economy, and a progressively inferior and deteriorating food and water supply, and the implications are virtually, if not wholly cataclysmic. The odds are clearly stacked against us.

How do we possibly overcome this?

Here's how:

First, we *must* take a keen interest in the "machine"—our primal body and mind—which we inhabit. We must strive to understand our own inner workings as much as humanly possible.

We must strive to apply what we know about the selective pressures over 100,000 generations that shaped our physiology to what we choose to eat.

We *must not* simply trust others to manage our health for us, especially where others' interests may not lie with our best interests but instead with profit.

We must avoid the temptation of "food as a source of cheap, nutrient-devoid entertainment" and, instead make conscious, deliberate and wise choices about what it is we mindfully incorporate into our living matrix.

We must do what our ancestors also did as they had to—we must adapt. We also are forced to take certain compensatory steps our ancestors didn't really need to take. One of the first orders of business in this adaptation is to compensate—as much as is possible—for the bombardment of toxic, oxidative onslaught from our environment. As such . . .

Our need for antioxidants has never been greater. Even though vegetables and greens were mostly an optional source of nutrients in our most primitive, Ice-Age past, the time has come to greatly increase their role in our modern diets—both to provide a varied plethora of phytonutrients and antioxidants to our beleaguered, embattled cells, and also, to some degree, to provide fiber as a means of binding unwanted conjugated, carcinogenic xenoestrogens and eliminating them from our bodies, preventing their reabsorption. Plant foods are probably more important to us now than ever.

We must avoid irradiated and/or chemically treated vegetables as much as possible by buying from local farmers, farmer's markets and co-ops, and/or growing your own. This should be a high priority.

Dietary supplements also have a role to play in supplying us with concentrated sources of key nutrients and antioxidants, both fat- and water-soluble. Depleted nutrients in our soils and other modern factors also make supplementation, to at least some degree, a modern necessity. Anti-glycating supplemental nutrients may also further slow the degenerative ravages of dietary glucose.

I also advocate the use of concentrated, unsweetened quality "green drinks" (powdered organic vegetable, leafy green and phytonutrient concentrates) as a means of getting more concentrated phyto-nutrition and providing a detoxifying and alkalinizing nutritional boost to otherwise nutrient-depleted produce from our nutrient-depleted soils.

This soil-depletion issue also makes the use of ionic trace mineral supplement complexes extremely valuable, if not essential, to ensure a complete source of trace elements necessary for innumerable cellular and bioelectric processes. "Trace Mineral Drops" by Trace Minerals Research and/or Himalayan or Celtic sea salt are all excellent means of supporting these dietary requirements.

A greatly increased need for quality (pure) hydration is also probable. Although our ancestors likely did not consume "eight full glasses of water per day" or carry around water bottles, the dehydrating tendencies of modern stress, diuretics (medication, high carbohydrate diets, gym workouts, caffeine, etc.), plus the excessive burden of toxicity in our bodies and in our environment, make this a much more sensible modern practice.

The burden of our overwhelmingly toxic environment and contaminated air, water and food supply also leads to a need for active and preferably multiple, varied and regular practices of detoxification. Physical movement such as exercise, good hydration, "green drinks," colon hydrotherapy, far infra-red saunas, rebounding (using mini-trampolines—outstanding exercise for improved lymphatic circulation), and even ten and twenty-one-day periodic detoxification programs designed by a qualified natural healthcare provider, or a Certified Nutritional Therapist/Nutritional Therapy Practitioner may be necessary and beneficial for many.

Minimizing the toxic burden on our tissues and eliminative organs and up-regulating their efficiency is key. Maintaining the up-regulation of our "repair and regeneration" mode by dietary optimization of carbohydrate, protein and fat macronutrients as described throughout this book is essential.

Finally, stress management practice today is absolutely mandatory. Fast-paced lifestyles, modern societal pressures, EMF pollution from cell phones, wi-fi, and other electrical contamination of our home environments affects us all.

There are any number of stress management techniques ranging from meditation, biofeedback or neurofeedback, to therapeutic massage that should be incorporated into the lives of literally everyone. This is not about luxury . . . it is about necessity.

We *must* accept responsibility for the health and function (and dysfunction) of our own primal bodies and minds, understanding that we ultimately control our own genetic destiny and to a very significant degree, our own quality *and* quantity of life.

We also need to become activists, and no longer simply complacently accept the standards for our health and food supply as established and maintained by the multi-national, mono-culture agricultural, food industry and medical, pharmaceutical, and other greed- and ignorance-driven corporate interests (or the "regulatory agencies" such as the FDA which coddles them).

Support the work of the Weston A. Price Foundation and other consumer advocate groups striving to make a difference. Buy locally produced real food and produce, shop local food cooperatives and farmer's markets as much as possible, rather than larger chain stores, and join CSA (Community Supported Agriculture) programs (see appendices for resources). Read Appendix A, too, for tips on just getting started.

It *is* possible to survive—and even thrive—in this modern world. It is possible to avoid the ravages of our nation's healthcare crisis and corrupt corporate manipulations . . . but only the uniquely-informed, educated, nutritionally disciplined and savvy are likeliest to do so.

That's a cold, hard reality.

We cannot afford to be ignorant any longer. We cannot afford not to care or be simply cynical. We cannot afford to blindly depend on a corrupt and broken "healthcare system" to save us. We cannot afford to take *anything* for granted.

We still possess all the potential for physical and mental excellence our primitive ancestors enjoyed—plus we now have the science and the awareness of how to use Mother Nature's agenda to our best advantage. We actually have the capacity and key information that can allow us to live longer and healthier than we ever have before in our long evolutionary history . . .

. . . but only if we have the wisdom to actually use it.

Men occasionally stumble over the truth, but most of them pick themselves up and hurry off as if nothing had happened.
—WINSTON CHURCHILL

APPENDIX A:
WHERE TO START?

Although the amount of information covered in this volume may seem a bit overwhelming (to say nothing of paradigm-shifting, for some), it does not have to be a complicated process getting started. Depending upon just how gung-ho you are willing to be, there are some simple steps one can take to get underway toward improved physical/mental health and well-being.

Step #1: **Become very conscious of food and beverage choices.** Ask yourself whether what you are eating is something that might have resembled "food" or nourishment to someone 40,000+ years ago (in the hey-day before the birth of the "food industry"). Ask yourself whether what you are eating is more likely to promote your health, or constitute "a backslide." Live consciously. Do not fear occasional indulgences, just make them occasional and be fully aware of the choices you make. **Read labels carefully!**

Step #2: **The closer you can come to eliminating all forms of sugar and starch (including grains, bread, pasta, rice, potatoes, desserts, juices, alcohol, honey, maple syrup . . . etc.)—by far the better.** I used to believe it was better to start by cutting the amount of carbs eaten in half, then gradually reducing the carbs further from there; but my clinical experience has overwhelmingly shown that it is far less painful and more effective to simply eliminate them and get your body used to the idea of using fat, rather than sugar, as its primary source of fuel as soon as possible. Until that time, your body will simply continue to depend on sugar as its primary source of fuel and you will still be subject to blood sugar's whims and fluctuations. This actually makes the successful transition to primary fat-burning much harder and you will likely continue to suffer cravings, weight loss resistance and other issues. Eliminating nearly all carbs (sources of sugar and starch) other than fibrous vegetables and all but very small amounts of fruit ASAP is the best possible goal. The use of supplements such as L-glutamine powder and/or gymnema sylvestre can serve as supplemental "training wheels" to help eliminate hypoglycemia issues or temporary cravings, while the use of L-carnitine can help more efficiently and rapidly facilitate the body's use of fat as its main source of fuel.

The results of going "cold turkey" with respect to carbohydrate elimination, combined with moderating protein intake and using fat to satisfy appetite can be quite surprisingly and dramatically positive in its effect and far easier than one might otherwise suspect. The liberation from unhealthy cravings and blood sugar roller-coaster-ing can feel like a nearly overnight miracle to some.

Step #3: **Eliminate margarine and vegetable shortening, as well as any commercial brands of cooking oil *immediately,* if not yesterday.** Buy extra virgin olive oil (organic, if possible), sesame oil, coconut oil, and organic or pasture-fed butter (raw butter from a local farm, if available). Avoid the use of any other commercial or even organic vegetable oils, as they contain excessive omega-6 and frequently contain trans fats. They are also very prone to rancidity. Rice bran oil, currently being used in many restaurants for high heat cooking as a means of avoiding trans fats is probably okay, though of no particular benefit.

Step #4: **Substitute Celtic or Himalayan sea salt for refined table salt.** It is an excellent full-spectrum source of trace elements (not just refined sodium) and it tastes much better!

Step #5: **Get rid of all the sodas, sports beverages and juices and focus on drinking pure, clean water.** Self-serve water dispensers are available at many markets and typically dispense high quality reverse-osmosis water that has been both carbon filtered and UV-sterilized at a minimal cost per gallon (25–35 cents). Better yet (and at ultimately far less cost-per gallon), install a high quality reverse osmosis water purification system in your own home (warning: you get what you pay for).

Step #6: **Avoid "fast-food" restaurants.** If you need a meal "in a pinch" you could try carrying some snacks along like jerky, pemmican, canned tuna, sardines or nuts (see snack list). If this isn't enough, then seek out natural foods-type delis for sliced, unprocessed lunch meats and salads (with simple olive oil and vinegar).

Step #7: **Begin shopping in more natural, organic, biodynamic-oriented and especially farmers markets. Buy locally grown produce.** Avoid the "center aisles," the pre-packaged, non-perishable section, and stick to fresh meats and produce. Check the Web site www.eatwild.com for local farms carrying grass-fed products (meats, eggs and dairy) and contact a local chapter of the Weston A. Price Foundation for the largest array of local resources. Frequently, members will pool their purchases with CSAs (Community Supported Agriculture programs), allowing for huge savings on meats and produce. It's also a great way to get free helpful advice and moral support (see www.WestonAPrice.org).

Step #8: **Begin supplementing with omega-3 oils.** Fish oil is vastly preferable to flax oil. More than a teaspoon or a tablespoon may be needed at first. With respect to capsules, the standard fish oil capsule contains around 180 mg of EPA and 120 mg of DHA. Recommended dosage for remediation of especially deficient states is about one capsule for every 10–15 pounds of body weight, preferably in two divided doses. Once symptoms and/or sense of well-being improve, cut back to smaller amounts, if desired. Flax oil can also be additionally beneficial in small amounts but should *not* constitute the sole source of omega-3 in the diet.

Individuals with learning disabilities, mood disorders or ADD/HD and those of Scandinavian, Northern European, Native American or Coastal Irish descent tend to lack the delta-6 desaturase enzyme necessary for proper conversions to the active derivative forms of EPA and DHA and *must* get these in animal/fish source forms.

Step #9: **Include a teaspoon or two for children, and at least one or two tablespoons for adults of high vitamin cod liver oil a day for a superior and reliable source of vitamins A and D.** The body cannot make adequate use of minerals or function optimally without these important fat-soluble nutrients, and diets today don't tend to provide adequate levels. Test periodically for vitamin D (25, hydroxy-D) levels in the blood.

Step #10: **Begin supplementing with a quality vitamin or mineral complex and/or a multi-mineral complex,** *amino acid* chelated preferably that includes particularly those minerals most deficient in soils and, consequently, diets: iodine, magnesium, zinc, selenium, manganese, chromium, boron, vanadium. The body can do little with vitamins without these and other minerals present, together with numerous trace elements. Trace elements are best supplemented by unrefined Celtic or Himalayan sea salt or by ionic Trace Mineral Drops, available in most health food stores. Reliable dietary sources of these trace elements are wild-caught seafood, and Celtic sea salt.

Please avoid colloidal minerals. If stress, immune, mood or cognitive dysfunction are an issue, adding extra water soluble nutrients such as vitamins B complex and C may be additionally advisable. If ADD/HD, depression, anxiety or immune dysfunction is an issue, additional zinc and/or magnesium (ionic, in solution, or amino acid chelate) may be important, if not essential.

Step #11: **Become physically active, preferably finding something you really enjoy.** It should not have to be overly strenuous or time consuming, but it should be something you can see yourself doing consistently. Some form of weight training and/or other forms of anaerobic activity (e.g., sprinting, "power walking") should be considered. No more than an hour or two per week *total* preferably broken up into roughly 3–5 separate days should be necessary to achieve desired results. Quality of time (that is, intensity) in the gym rather than quantity is key with weights. Weights and other anaerobic challenge give far more bang for the buck than "aerobics" for weight loss and improved cardio-pulmonary health. Weight training enhances growth hormone release (which burns fat and builds muscle) and improves metabolic efficiency via increases in lean tissue mass and increased mitochondrial density (our cell's fat burning factories). No more than about five minutes of aerobics—strictly as a warm-up—should be done on the same day as a weight-training workout, for best results. Do other forms of intense anaerobic-type exercise on the off-days apart from weight training. Additional time spent walking or cycling daily is fine.

Exercise improves insulin and leptin sensitivity and can improve cardio-pulmonary function . . . but remember that *too much* exercise can work against you.

Step #12: **Start exploring some of the references and Web sites provided in order to further educate and inspire your progress.** Don't take my word for it! Continuing education is hugely reinforcing and utterly key to long-term health.

Step #13: **If food allergies or sensitivities are suspected, then** spending no less than a week or two eliminating a suspected food from the diet may be a good way to find out whether it is to blame or not. Grains, soy, corn, peanuts, chicken eggs and dairy are the most likely place to start (not surprising, since they are post-agricultural foods, containing foreign proteins). Sensitivity to particularly grains (gluten) and dairy (casein) can also precipitate other sensitivities and allergic responses to other things over time, not to mention autoimmune disorders. Sticking to high quality protein from a variety of meats and/or seafood and vegetables/greens for a week is a worthwhile first step in finding whether symptoms improve. Further testing by a competent practitioner specializing in this issue may be necessary.

Step #14: **Become aware of the pervasive influence of EMF (electromagnetic frequency) pollution and take steps to protect yourself from its influence and do what you can nutritionally and stress-reduction-wise to help compensate for unavoidable exposure.** Minimize exposure to cordless phones and wi-fi routers, high tension power lines and cell phone radiation by taking precautionary measures (such as the utilization of "blue-tube"—*not* Bluetooth—type headsets for cell phones or using speaker phone options) or by eliminating these influences from your home and work environment as much as possible. Sleep environment is the most important, and unplugging electrical devices in your bedroom at night can greatly improve the quality of rest and regeneration you get from sleep. Get an old-fashioned battery-operated alarm clock. You can explore your own potential exposure to cell phone tower radiation by going to www.antennasearch.com.

Prepare to be blown away. I, personally, discovered 67 cell towers less than 4 miles from my home.

Step #15: **Be sure to get a minimum of 7–8 hours quality sleep every night. Be consistent!** Sleep deprivation (less than 6 hours a night) can lead to insulin resistance and hormonal dysregulation, as well as increased risk for cancer. Be sure the room you sleep in is as dark as possible (no night lights), or wear a soft eye mask. Unplug electrical devices in the bedroom and avoid carbohydrates, including alcohol, before bed, as this can result in sleep disturbances and night-time waking. Becoming a "fat burner" rather than a "sugar burner" will ultimately remove blood sugar fluctuations from the day- and nighttime-equation and allow for deeper, more restful and regenerative sleep.

Step #16: **Be sure to hydrate with pure, reverse-osmosis or contaminant-free water.** The rule of thumb here is to calculate half of your body weight in pounds and consume roughly that amount in ounces of pure, fresh and clean water per day. Don't exceed 100 ounces a day, though. Too much is as undesirable as too little.

Step #17: **Practice stress reduction and detoxification regularly, if not daily.** Saunas (especially *far infra-red*), green drinks, the use of chlorella (to aid in detoxification of heavy metals), proper hydration, exercise, skin brushing and/or rebounding (for enhanced lymphatic drainage), meditation, biofeedback, attitude awareness, and cultivation of positive and constructive emotional states should all be practiced by everyone. Periodically, more intensive detoxification measures such as colon hydrotherapy and/or carefully designed 21-day detox programs, should be considered good, sound preventative medicine. Our bodies and minds need all the help they can get to overcome the burdens of our toxic environment and food supply!

Step #18: **Create or find a health or nutritional support group.** Joining the Weston A. Price Foundation and/or attending WAPF potlucks can be fun, educational and a great source of feedback and support. Subscribing to the *Primal Body—Primal Mind* Web site (www. PrimalBody-PrimalMind.com) and newsletter can keep you "in the loop" with new findings, support and reminders about how to lead a healthier life. Finding friends and family members willing to join in your efforts is essential for long-term success in creating the kind of health you want and deserve. There are too many counter-productive influences in our environment and in the media to "go it alone."

Step #18: **Try (ideally) to incorporate at least 50% of combined animal (yes, animal) and vegetable source foods in your diet as raw or minimally cooked and/or cultured.** The USDA says that meat or fish that has been frozen solid for two weeks is safe from parasitic concerns for raw consumption. Safety guidelines, quality meat and fish sources and careful preparation here are important, so be careful . . . but raw and cultured foods have many important benefits that are readily lost to cooking. Marinades made with lemon juice, liquid whey and vinegars also help minimize risks associated with raw meat or fish. Taking hydrochloric acid tablets with meals containing raw meat and/or fish may also provide a certain degree of reliable protection from food born illness. Salads, raw fibrous veggies, microgreens, sprouts, lacto-fermented vegetables, raw-milk yogurt and kefir, raw-milk pastured cheeses, butter, tartars, raw egg yolks from pastured eggs, Carpaccio, sashimi, ceviches and lox all possess potentially tremendous health benefits. These include vital nutrients, hydrophilic colloids, more easily-digested undenatured proteins, fresh non-rancid natural fats and oils, heat labile C and B vitamins, enzymes and/or probiotic cultures which not only improve the digestibility of these foods, but are immensely beneficial and nourishing in ways cooked foods can never be. This will be a stretch for some, especially where raw protein sources are concerned, but well worth the effort toward gradual incorporation into the diet.

"Raw foodists" (typically vegan) have it only partly right. *Exclusively* raw vegetable diets really only meet a partial need and raw veggies, although very cleansing to the system, are less digestible to us raw (seeing as we lack four stomachs), due to cellulose binding of many inherent nutrients. Also, many nutrients in vegetables (i.e., carotenoids), require dietary fat for proper assimilation. Juicing them is not the answer, either (see the chapter on juicing). Although one might initially feel fabulous on such a diet, as detoxifying and therapeutic short-term as it may be, it cannot be sustainable long term for optimal health.

Cleansing is *not* the same as rebuilding and adequately nourishing.

APPENDIX B:
SAMPLE MENUS

The following assumes organic, biodynamic and free-range or grass-fed wherever possible.

BREAKFAST: Duck or (if tolerated) chicken eggs, preferably boiled, poached or cooked sunny-side up, on low heat in butter keeping the yolks soft (scrambling eggs can oxidize the cholesterol contained in the yolks and is best not done too frequently). Poached eggs can be served with a bit of salmon, if desired. Stick to no more than an ounce or two of protein per meal. Use butter, olive oil or full-fat cheese (if tolerated) as needed to satisfy appetite.

Breakfast meats can include freshly ground sausage (many delicious varieties can be found at the meat counters of natural foods-type markets), small 2–3 oz steak, freshly ground beef or lamb with vegetables of choice (i.e., onions, mushrooms, spinach, broccoli, etc.). Breakfast can also be done with quick stir-frys or evening leftovers.

Who says breakfast has to look like "breakfast"?

Drink water, tea or small amounts of organic decaf coffee (in order of preference). Please avoid all juices, even organic.

LUNCH: Soups, salads with broiled meats or fish and homemade dressing made with: extra virgin olive oil, prepared mustard (read labels carefully!), and balsamic vinegar blended together—*delicious!* Sliced (not processed) meats and/or full-fat cow, sheep or goat raw milk cheeses with veggies, tuna salad (without the pasta), egg salad (without the potatoes), etc.

DINNER: Steak, roasts, lamb chops, fresh ground burgers without the bun, roast chicken, duck, turkey, ground meat (beef, lamb, venison) hash with veggies, ribs, stir frys, meatloaf (without breadcrumbs), broiled or sauteed salmon, halibut, tuna, escolar, mackerel, red snapper (with garlic butter), scallops, shrimp, stews without potatoes, casseroles without the noodles, hearty soups or large salads containing meat or seafood. *Again, stick to no more than 2–3 oz of meat or fish per serving, accompanied by various complements.* You'll be shocked by how much money you save and how satisfying this little protein can be. Trust me. I was.

Complements can include: sautéed mushrooms or onions, most any non-starchy vegetable such as broccoli, cauliflower, asparagus, snap peas, cabbage, brussel sprouts, or greens such as salads, or spinach, chard or kale sautéed with butter, olive or sesame oil. Pine nuts, walnuts, crushed hazelnuts or slivered almonds can be used as a garnish. M-m-good!

Nutritious Snack Foods
(or quick, healthy small meals "on the go")
- Raw nuts (that have preferably first been soaked overnight in salt water, drained, rinsed and dried in a 150 degree oven to eliminate phytates and trypsin inhibitors) including: macadamia, almonds, pecans, hazelnuts, brazil nuts, pumpkin seeds, walnuts, etc. Organic dry roasted and salted nuts are also acceptable.
- Nora's Nut Ball snackers (*oooh la-la!*)—see next page for recipe!
- Hard-boiled or deviled eggs (preferably organic, free-range)

- Sardines packed in olive oil (very rich in zinc and omega-3)
- Tuna packed in olive oil
- Tuna or chicken salad (w/o any macaroni)
- Sliced, seasoned avocado
- A slice or plain spoonful of pate (no crackers—except maybe Lydia's Organics brand—or bread!)
- A plain slice of grass-fed liverwurst or braunschweiger sausage (see U.S. Wellness Meats or www.grasslandbeef.com)
- Olives
- Cream cheese balls, herbed or plain, with an olive center (very tasty!)—credit and kudos to my wonderful, tastefully creative friend, Tina Gilbertson!
- Coconut flakes (*Bob's Red Mill* and *Living Tree Community Foods* brands have delicious packaged coconut in larger flakes)
- Green drinks (try *NanoGreens* ... great taste!)—incredible anti-oxidant content and very detoxifying
- Almond, or other nut butter—preferably not peanut or cashew butter (dip celery sticks or just a spoon into the jar and eat!)
- Plain organic, *whole-fat, homemade, raw milk* yogurt or kefir with berries or bee pollen granules
- Organic full-fat cheese slices (preferably raw milk based) or a slice of brie (goat and/or sheep milk) cheese may be substituted in many cases where casein sensitivity is an issue
- Homemade salmon jerky, beef jerky or pemmican (see recipes in *Nourishing Traditions* by Sally Fallon) or a good homemade-style beef jerky sold at a natural foods-type meat counter
- Raw veggies and homemade avocado dip or guacamole
- Thinly sliced turkey or roast beef rolled up with cheese or cream cheese
- Lox or smoked salmon—with or without cream cheese
- Shrimp cocktail with lemon

Dessert, Anyone (if you must)?

- Fresh berries of any variety alone, with fresh cream or blended with coconut milk and a pinch of Stevia
- Sliced fruit

Great Healthy Snack Food Recipe

Nora's Nut-Ball Snackers (I hope these aren't my only legacy)

The following recipe is for a snack many of my clients have fallen in love with. It's easy to make and utterly delicious. It's also very satisfying for both the taste buds and the appetite. Should you find yourself hungry between meals and need "a little something," I think you'll agree these are wonderful.

You'll need:

- One regular-sized jar of almond butter or any other nut butter—other than peanut or cashew butter—that you prefer. Stir surface oil in well!
- 10 oz. (a very rough approximation) of organic nuts (almonds, pecans, macadamias, brazil nuts, pistachios, etc.) preferably pre-soaked and dried. Use a food processor to grind or chop to desired consistency/"chunkiness."
- Handful of organic sesame seeds and/or chia seeds (great source of mucilaginous fiber to help "keep that train rolling").
- Organic shredded coconut (as much or as little as you like)
- Alcohol-free (glycerin-based) vanilla extract or crushed/powdered organic vanilla beans.
- One full brick (room temperature) of KerryGold butter (decidedly a "key" ingredient)

Optional ingredients:

- Organic coconut flour (*Bob's Red Mill* makes a good one)—add for additional yummy coconut flavor and/or better binding

- Organic coconut butter ... (you have to taste this stuff to believe it!)
- Stevia (for added sweetness, if needed or desired)
- Bee pollen (why not? Good source of flavinoids)
- Organic cacao nibs (*Dagoba* has quality ones)—adds chocolaty flavor without adding sugar. Also, cacao nibs have roughly two times the antioxidant content of green tea!
- Whatever floats your boat (and happens to be low carb)

Blend the above in a bowl thoroughly, then spoon out into little "balls" onto wax paper on a plate or tray. Refrigerate for a good hour, or until these firm up.

If you want to take them with you, you might consider placing them in a small portable cooler. You could also individually wrap these in wax paper to secure them (if they can't be refrigerated) so that they don't get all over everything if they melt.

Prepare your taste buds to be dazzled!

APPENDIX C:
AN ABBREVIATED GUIDE TO
SUPPLEMENTATION

Supplements, to begin with, are merely that: *supplemental* to a solid foundational diet. Numerous studies of primitive people groups have consistently shown a much greater nutrient density and vitamin/mineral contents many times what are typically consumed in foods today (see the table illustration earlier entitled "Average Contemporary Hunter-Gatherer Nutrient Intake").

Given the mineral depletion of our soils and the difficulty in obtaining adequate levels of essential fats and fat-soluble nutrients from readily available food sources, greater chronic levels of daily stress and environmental toxins, it stands to reason that some supplementation is desirable, if not necessary. Logically, it is best to obtain supplements from food sources or complexes wherever available, as numerous, possibly unidentified co-factors are likely to be present and help facilitate optimal utilization of the nutrients. For instance, add extra B complex via added nutritional (not "brewers") yeast as a condiment (yields a cheesy, nutty flavor). Bee pollen can serve as a source of healthy flavinoids. A teaspoon or two for a child to a tablespoon or two for an adult a day of high vitamin cod liver oil (www.greenpasture.org) is a wonderful and important way to add natural vital A and D, as well as small amounts of omega-3 to the diet.

Celtic or Himalayan sea salt and/or ionic Trace Mineral Drops by Trace Minerals Research can be a wonderfully reliable means of getting adequate trace elements in one's diet that are frequently missing from soils our food is grown in. A quality food-source multi-vitamin or mineral complex, too, can be helpful for some. I generally avoid most popular and/or generic supermarket and pharmacy brands (e.g., One-A-Day®, Centrum® . . . etc.). Please be aware of labels and, more specifically, additives commonly found in most commercial supplements. "Magnesium Stearate" and/or "Stearic acid" are unnecessary additives and most sources contain trans fats. Studies by the University of Texas Health Science Center and the East Carolina University School of Medicine reveal that these toxic excipients cause a rapid collapse of T-cell membrane function and cell death, therefore suppressing the immune system (*Immunology*, 1990, Jul.).

Also, "When cells were exposed to stearic acids and palmitic acids, there was a dramatic loss of cell viability after 24 hours. Cell death was induced by stearic and palmitic acid" (Ulloth).

Not the kind of stuff you'd expect to find in a *health food* supplement.

Another additive of concern is titanium dioxide, which "rapidly damages neurons at low concentrations in complex brain cultures" (Long et al, 2007). Also, titanium dioxide has recently been classified by the International Agency for Research on Cancer (IARC) as an IARC Group 2B carcinogen "possibly carcinogenic to humans" (Canadian Centre for Occupational Health and Safety). This substance is also widely used in cosmetics and sun-block lotions. In addition, it has been strongly linked to autoimmune conditions (Dietrich Klinghardt, MD, PhD). Just because you find a supplement in a health food store (or pharmacy) does not automatically make it healthy for you. *Always* read labels, including "other ingredients."

Finding supplemental sources that avoid magnesium stearate or stearic acid, or titanium dioxide, although challenging, can also improve bioavailability of vitamins, minerals and other nutrients/supplements purchased. Additive-free supplements are typically available from healthcare providers almost exclusively, but there are exceptions. Also, see resources in Appendix F.

In some cases there may be pronounced deficiency states of certain nutrients, as with many cases of ADD/HD and other learning disabilities. In these cases, supplement with extra ionic zinc, ionic magnesium, B complex, cod liver oil (to improve mineral absorption and utilization), and omega-3 fish oil. Initially, more of some nutrients may be needed to make up the deficits.

A list of some supplements worthy of general consideration follows. Not everyone will need all of these, but depending on your state of health and ability to afford quality supplements, many of these may be worthwhile. My focus is with commonly deficient or easily depleted nutrients, antioxidants and anti-glycating substances.

- Omega-3 fish oil caps: Roughly 2,000mg/day may be adequate for basic health maintenance or cognitive enhancement. Where weight problems, mood or learning disorders are an issue, higher doses starting with one standard capsule per each ten pounds of body weight—preferably in two divided doses, may be needed to remediate deficiency (Mercola 2002). Up to 10,000 mg/day may be required in cases of more serious mood disorders or bipolar disorder (Stoll 1998). In these cases, use liquid preparations rather than capsules. *Note:* Some dietary saturated fat is necessary for both protection and proper utilization of these delicate essential oils, along with supplemental vitamins D and E.
- Cod Liver Oil: 1–2 *tsp* for children or 1–2 *tbs*+ for adults

- Vitamin E, rich in gamma tocopherols: 400–800 IU daily (aids in protection and metabolism of delicate EFAs)
- Selenium (from Selenomethionene)—200–400 mcg daily (required for optimal utilization of vitamin E)
- B-complex—take with every meal. B-vitamins are commonly lost with stress and diuretics, as well as carbohydrate consumption
- B12 (Methylcobalamin): 1–5 mg per day as a sublingual liquid or lozenge. Is needed for healthy brain function as well as the manufacture of red blood cells, cardiovascular health and numerous other critical functions. Many have inadequate or deficient levels and have digestive issues that make the absorption of B12 from food difficult
- Complexed vitamin C: be sure the vitamin C you take is complexed with other co-factors (bioflavinoids). Taking "ascorbic acid" alone can lead to a depletion of other cofactors that ultimately prevents proper utilization of ascorbic acid
- Ascorbyl palmitate: the fat soluble form of vitamin C that is able to actually cross cellular membranes and perform antioxidant and anti-glycating protection *within* the cell, where nuclear material and mitochondria lie
- CoQ10 50–100mg for adults, if affordable (adds additional protection to EFAs and enhances mitochondrial function. A potent antioxidant)
- Black Currant Seed Oil or Evening Primrose Oil (sources of GLA): Follow dosage recommendations on bottle
- Also refer back to chapter on blood glucose regulation for supplements aiding insulin/leptin sensitivity and anti-glycation

Eventually, getting most things from the highest quality food sources should be the ultimate goal, though for some may not always be practical or feasible. Given our modern agricultural practices, modern lifestyles, the prevalence of toxins in our environment, and the occasional difficulty in obtaining the best quality foods from un-adulterated sources it is realistic to expect some necessary ongoing supplementation for optimal health.

It is wise to be mindful that the extra investment in quality food and supplementation *now* is vastly preferable to dependence on medi-cations (which only treat symptoms and harbor side effects), surgery and hospitalization down the road. In the end, costs of these negative consequences extend far beyond the mere financial.

What good is quantity of life without real quality?

Furthermore, the proper foundational support provided by opti-mal diet and supplementation, as well as the development, nurturing and well-being of a child's developing mind and body cannot be ig-nored or left to chance in this modern, corporate-predatory world.

APPENDIX D:
THE WESTON A. PRICE FOUNDATION

D r. Weston Price, a prominent dentist and respected scientist in the early 1900s noticed that, between the years of 1910 and 1925, children of his dental patients had problems their parents never had. He noticed an emerging pattern of crowded, crooked or missing teeth and malformed dental arches. (In fact, orthodontia was developed around this time for treating this widespread newly emerging problem.) Dr. Price looked to primitive cultures, long renowned for their splendid, beautiful teeth and physical excellence and wondered whether there was something present in their native diets that might account for this. He also questioned what effect modernization and refinement of foods might be having on many primitive societies newly adopting the emerging Western diet.

It was a truly unique era where air travel had only begun to make far reaches of the globe accessible in a way they never had before. And yet, the tentacles of civilization had not yet reached much of it. Numerous primitive and traditional societies were still thriving in ways they had for hundreds, thousands or tens of thousands of years. It was a window of opportunity unlike any other in history. Dr. Price saw this and, enviably, took full advantage of it.

Over the next ten years both Weston Price and his wife traveled over 100,000 miles studying numerous primitive and/or traditional societies, among them Swiss villagers in remote mountain valleys,

South Pacific Islanders, Aborigines, peoples of remote Celtic isles, African tribes throughout the African continent, American Indians, Innuit (Eskimos) and many others. He noticed that all primitive and traditional groups studied typically had all thirty-two teeth, perfectly fitting dental arches and perfectly formed teeth, suffering little or no decay, as long as they had no access to modern foods. Where cultural and dietary integration to modern lifestyle had begun to occur, he noticed first dental decay and systemic disease, then the emergence of crooked, malformed teeth and dental arches, as well as narrowed or malformed facial features in subsequent generations. He also noted a direct correlation between the health of an individual's teeth and gums and overall health and resistance to disease.

Dr. Price sent back to laboratories and analyzed more than ten thousand samples of native foods. Price's analysis revealed that those on native diets consumed more than ten-times of the many then-known vitamins and minerals than those eating modern refined foods. Especially significant were very high levels of fat-soluble, animal source vitamins A and D—frequently 10 times the current RDAs. For many other nutrients the figure was as much as 30, 40—*even 50 times more* than found in modern diets.

Clearly, the implications are staggering. And these peoples suffered almost none of the many diseases that were then plaguing Western civilization. He also noted several significant common factors among the diets of each of these unique cultures that he believed accounted for consistently superior health, physical structure and astonishing freedom from disease. Particularly notable was the central importance of animal source foods and richly abundant fat-soluble nutrients in all cultures studied. He was unable to find a single vegetarian primitive society anywhere in the world out of hundreds, to his own considerable disappointment.

He published a book by the title: *Nutrition and Physical Degeneration,* in 1939, which chronicled in exhaustively documented scientific detail and photographs the findings of his journeys to the remote corners of the globe in search for the answers to health and disease. This book was required reading for many years in Harvard anthropology classes. It just may be the most important work on diet and health ever written.

Today, the Weston A. Price Foundation is a nonprofit, tax-exempt charity founded in 1999 to disseminate the research of nutrition pioneer Weston A. Price, DDS. The foundation is dedicated to restoring nutrient-dense foods to the American diet through education, research and activism and supports a number of movements that contribute to this objective, including: accurate nutrition instruction, organic and biodynamic farming, pasture feeding of livestock, community supported farms, honest and informative labeling, prepared parenting and nurturing therapies. Specific goals of the foundation include establishment of universal access to clean, certified raw milk and a ban on the use of soy formula for infants.

Numerous chapters are currently active throughout the country and may be found via the Web site: www.WestonAPrice.org. Local chapters can be an invaluable source for locating quality sources of grass-fed meats, and dairy products, as well as biodynamically-grown vegetables and free-range eggs. Regular meetings often highlight presentations or potlucks, and provide a supportive environment, as well as great recipes and tips, for individuals and families seeking a healthier way to live. One does not need to be a member in most cases to attend.

.

APPENDIX E:
PYROLURIA

Pyroluria is a little known but not entirely uncommon genetic condition affecting roughly 11% of the population. People with pyroluria produce excess amounts of a byproduct from hemoglobin synthesis, called OHHPL (hydroxyhemoppyrrolin-2-one), an otherwise unimportant waste product. Significantly elevated levels of OHHPL, however, bind excessively to zinc and B6 leading to potentially severe deficiencies of these important nutrients. Pyroluria is diagnosed by the presence of elevated *kryptopyrroles* (KP) in the urine.

The diagnosis is widely recognized within the field of orthomolecular medicine and orthomolecular psychiatry but little acknowledged within conventional medical circles. The pyroluria diagnosis and hypothesis has also been strongly acknowledged and advocated, by Carl Pfieffer of Emory University, and the Princeton Brain-Bio Center, a precursor of the Pfieffer Treatment Center.

In normal individuals, KP are simply a waste product created from the production of hemoglobin, which are typically just excreted and of no significant biological consequence. In pyrolurics, however, these metabolites cannot be excreted and they then bind relentlessly with zinc and B6, making them unavailable to the body to a greater or lesser degree, depending on the severity of the condition. This, of course, is extremely problematic and has all sorts of negative and profound implications for neurotransmitter production, immune functioning, cognitive functioning, digestion and a few hundred or so other things. The effects can be anywhere from mild to severe. Stress tends to elevate kryptopyrroles levels and their impact in these individuals. If left untreated, this can lead to a wide variety of fairly significant and mounting health problems.

Regular physicians rarely test for this and, in fact, may know little about it or may even deny the validity of the disorder, as there are no drugs to treat it. Nonetheless, it is becoming increasingly well known and screened for among alternative healthcare providers and nutritional management may offer profound relief for many that was not achievable any other way. Nutritional management of pyroluria, once properly diagnosed, generally involves relatively large doses of zinc and B6, as well as added GLA (gamma-linolenic acid) supplementation (i.e., black currant seed oil) and diets higher in arachidonic acid.

Pyroluria is fairly commonly associated with a number of disorders, including depression, anxiety spectrum disorders, autism, Tourette's, bipolar disorder, intractable mood disorders, immune problems, chronic acne, eczema, psoriasis, alcoholism and others. Pyrolurics also tend, in general, to be fairly stress-intolerant.

In formal clinical trials, the following percentages were determined for the occurrence of Pyroluria in various disorders:

▸ Autism: 50% (Audha)
▸ Alcoholism: 40% (Mathews-Larson)
▸ Schizophrenia: 70% (Hoffer)
▸ Depression: 70% (Hoffer)
▸ ADHD: 30% (Walsh)

Pyroluria may be readily diagnosed with a simple, inexpensive test, designed to detect abnormal kryptopyrolles in the urine. Normal results are typically less than 10 mcg/dL of KP. Borderline pyroluria may exist between 10–20mcg/dL (assess symptoms) and may respond nicely to aforementioned nutritional support. Anything over 20mcg/dL—particularly when coupled with symptoms—is considered full-blown pyroluria.

Although the diagnosis may be considered "controversial" by conventional medical standards, the clinical effects of proper nutritional support tend to be undeniable and can be quite dramatic. Testing and (when appropriate) nutritional support in symptomatic individuals are well worth the exploration.

Pyroluria and borderline pyroluria is readily manageable with high doses of zinc and B6 (and some extra GLA)—and that's the really good news. The downside of this is that supplementation must be life long in order to successfully manage the condition. It is especially important that the zinc be in a *highly* absorbable, readily bioavailable form (not tablets). For these purposes, I tend to recommend ionic forms of pure zinc—not blended with other minerals—in liquid solution (see resources in Appendix F). The results of appropriate supplementation in milder cases can be dramatic and profound for some, though in more severe cases improvement may be more gradual over three to twelve months.

Testing for this condition is simple, relatively inexpensive and readily accessible to anyone without a prescription. Contact Bio Center Lab in Wichita, Kansas (Phone: 316-684-7784 or 1-800-494-7785). Here is their Web site for more information: http://brightspot.org/biocenter.

A Few Symptoms and Characteristics Commonly Associated with Pyroluria (Testing may be worthwhile if a third or more of these symptoms apply to you)

- Little or no dream recall
- White spots on finger nails
- Poor morning appetite +/- tendency to skip breakfast
- Morning nausea
- Pale skin +/- poor tanning +/- burn easy in sun
- Sensitivity to bright light
- Hypersensitive to loud noises

- Reading difficulties (e.g. dyslexia)
- Poor ability to cope with stress
- Mood swings or temper outbursts
- Histrionic (dramatic) tendency
- Argumentative/enjoy argument
- Much higher capability and alertness in the evening, compared to mornings
- Poor short term memory
- Abnormal body fat distribution
- Dry skin
- Anxiousness
- Reaching puberty later than normal
- Difficulty digesting, a dislike of protein or a history of vegetarianism
- Tendency toward being a loner and/or avoiding larger groups of people
- Stretch marks on skin (continued)
- Poor sense of smell or taste
- A tendency to overreact to tranquilizers, barbiturates, alcohol or other drugs (in other words, a little produces a powerful response)
- A tendency toward anemia
- History of mental illness or alcoholism in family
- Easily upset by criticism
- Sweet smell (fruity odor) to breath or sweat when ill or stressed
- Prone to acne, eczema or psoriasis
- A tendency toward feeling anxious, fearful and carrying lifelong inner tension
- Difficulty recalling past events or people
- Bouts of depression or nervous exhaustion
- Prone to frequent colds or infections

APPENDIX F:
PALEO/TRADITIONAL DIET
RESOURCES AND RELATED WEB SITES

Primal Body-Primal Mind—a cutting edge educational and informational resource: www.PrimalBody-PrimalMind.com

Nutritional Therapy Association (NTA)—A unique and excellent source of certified education in nutritional therapy with an emphasis on physiology, human evolutionary history, and the work of numerous acclaimed nutritional pioneers: www.NutritionalTherapy.com

Weston A. Price Foundation

www.WestonAPrice.org

Price-Pottenger Nutrition Foundation

www.Price-Pottenger.org

Paleolithic Diet Page

www.PaleoDiet.com

Paleolithic Diet and Exercise Symposium Archive

http://maelstrom.stjohns.edu/archives/paleodiet.html

Paleofood: real world experiences of people trying to follow Paleolithic-based (hunter-gatherer) diets: http://maelstrom.stjohns.edu/archives/paleofood.html

Beyond Vegetarianism: An investigative Web site containing some excellent scientific research relating to Paleo diets: www.beyondveg.com

"The Paleolithic Diet and its Modern Implications: An Interview with Loren Cordain, PhD," by Robert Crayhon, MS www.lifeservices.com/cordain.htm

"Cereal Grains: Humanity's Double-Edged Sword" by Loren Cordain, PhD: A scientific paper on the history and health risks of grains with 342 scientific references: http://dfhi.com/interviews/cordaingrain/cordaingrain.html

EnteroLab—A fully accredited and registered lab specializing in testing for common food sensitivities. Extremely accurate testing and a superb resource for information: www.enterolab.com

The Gluten Free-Casein Free Web Site—Addresses issues of learning disabilities, ADD/HD, autism and other health issues as related to grain and commercial dairy products in the diet: www.gfcfdiet.com

Doctor Mercola, MD's Web Site—Filled with hundreds of diet and health-related articles, many elaborating on the topics of low carbohydrate diets, Paleo diets, soy dangers, etc. Free subscription to e-newsletter available. Very worthwhile: www.Mercola.com

Eat Wild—An entire Web site devoted to extolling the many benefits of pasture-fed vs. grain-fed meat—very educational. Also lists a nationwide directory of places where quality range-fed meat, poultry and eggs may be purchased. An invaluable resource! www.eatwild.com

The Truth about Soy—Exhaustively referenced throughout and detailed: www.soyonlineservice.co.nz

Native Foods—Explore Dr. Weston Price's research, *Nourishing Traditions,* and how to integrate them into your daily life through connection with this online forum: http://www.onelist.com/community/native-nutrition

A Campaign for Real Milk—Information regarding unpasteurized or unhomogenized (raw) milk products and available sources: www.realmilk.com

Radiant Life—a catalog of quality *Nourishing Traditions*-related products, supplements and foods: www.4radiantlife.com

Green Pasture—a superb source for high vitamin cod liver oil and high vitamin butter oil: www.greenpasture.org

Dr. Ron F. Schmid's Web site—a source of quality additive-free supplements available to everyone. Highly recommended! Tell Dr. Ron that Nora sent you ☺: www.drrons.com

Ionic Zinc and Magnesium liquid source—MMI laboratories, Inc., 1-888 775-7456 or www.ionicmagnesium.com

U.S. Wellness Meats—online mail order source of superb, organic grass-fed meats:www.grasslandbeef.com

Cholesterol Skeptics—www.thincs.org—a non-commercial organization of doctors and scientists providing information opposing the prevalent dogma about cholesterol and heart disease.

Resources for identifying hidden sources of MSG: www.truthinlabeling.org/hiddensources.html and www.truthinlabeling.org/addendum.html

microwavenews.com—definitive source of research information and news concerning the effects of EMF

LessEMF.com—source of emf-protective products

RFSafe.com—source of emf-protective products

APPENDIX G:
PROTEIN CONTENT IN FOODS

Sources: USDA Nutrient Database for Standard Reference

Complete Sources (note that amount of protein varies with fat content. More fat=less protein per serving). The following are approximations.

Based on a 3 ounce serving:

- Eggs (medium): 6 grams
- Fish (3 oz): 21 grams
- Cheese (cheddar): 25 grams
- Roast beef: 28 grams
- Roast chicken: 25 grams
- Other meats (avg): 25 grams
- Sausages: 12 grams
- Ham: 18 grams
- Beef burgers: 20 grams
- Corned beef: 26 grams
- Liver: 23 grams
- Sirloin steak: 24
- Turkey: 25 grams
- Shrimp: 18–21 grams
- Tuna: 22 grams
- Ground beef (regular): 23 grams
- Ground beef (lean): 24 grams
- Spareribs (lean): 22 grams

- ▸ Chicken breast: 25 grams
- ▸ Lobster: 17 grams
- ▸ Salmon: 22 grams
- ▸ Feta cheese: 12 grams
- ▸ Duck (roasted): 24 grams
- ▸ Whole milk yogurt (8oz): 7 grams

Protein Content in Incomplete or Plant Sources of Foods
(Even though incomplete protein, these foods contribute to the amino acid pool and thus may influence mTOR):

- ▸ Nuts (walnuts, brazil nuts) ¼ cup: 5 grams
- ▸ Cashews (1/4 cup): 5 grams
- ▸ Peanuts (1/4 cup): 9.5 grams
- ▸ Peanut butter (2 tbs): 8 grams
- ▸ Almonds (1/4 cup): 7.5 grams
- ▸ Pine nuts (1/4 cup): 7.5 grams
- ▸ Sunflower seeds (1/4 cup): 6.5 grams
- ▸ Oatmeal (1 cup): 6 grams
- ▸ Black beans (1/4 cup): 4.5 grams
- ▸ Pinto beans (1/4 cup): 3.5 grams
- ▸ Chick peas (1/4 cup): 4 grams
- ▸ Hummus: 5 grams
- ▸ Tabbouli: (3 oz) 3 grams
- ▸ Quinoa (1/2 cup): 4.5 grams
- ▸ Lentils (1.2 cup): 9 grams
- ▸ Tempeh (1/2 cup): 20 grams
- ▸ Brown rice (1/2 cup): 2.5 grams
- ▸ Stir-fried vegetables (1/2 cup): 2 grams
- ▸ Broccoli (1/2 cup): 2.5–3 grams)
- ▸ Spinach (1/2 cup): 2.5 grams
- ▸ Coconut milk (1 cup): 6 grams

REFERENCES

Paleolithic Diet/Protein/Mtor

Books:

Ardrey, R. 1976. *The hunting hypothesis*. New York, NY: Bantam.

Audette, R. and T. Gilchrist. 1999. Foreward to *NeanderThin* by M. Eades, MD. New York: St. Martin's Press.

Bronowski, J. 1974. *Ascent of man*. Boston: Little Brown and Co.

Cordain, L., PhD. 2002, *The Paleo diet* New York: John Wiley & Sons, Inc.

Crawford, M. and M. David. "Nutrition and evolution

Crayhon, R., MS. 1998. *Carnitine miracle*. NewYork: M. Evans & Company, Inc.

Crayhon, R., MS. 1994. *Nutrition made simple,* New York: M. Evans and Company, Inc.

Diamond, J. 1992. *The third chimpanzee: the evolution and future of the human animal*. HarperCollins.

Eades, M., MD, and Mary Dan Eades, MD. 2000. *The protein power lifeplan: a new comprehensive blueprint for optimal health*. New York: Warner Books, Inc.

Harris, M. and E.B. Ross, eds. *Food and evolution: toward a theory of human food habits.*

Hunt, C. 1999. Foreward to *Diet evolution* by M. and M.D. Eades, MDs. Maximum Human Potential Productions.

Leakey, R.E. and L. Roger.1977. *Origins: The emergence and evolution of our species and its possible future*. New York: EP Dutton.

Lindeberg, S. 2005. "Palaeolithic diet," *Scandinavian Journal of Food & Nutrition,* 49.2: 75–77.

Peskin, B., professor emeritus. 2001. *Peak performance—radiant health: moving beyond the zone*. Houston, TX: Noble Publishing.

Price, W., DDS. 1989. *Nutrition and physical degeneration*. New Canaan, Connecticut: Keats Publishing. (originally published, 1945, 1970.)

Schmid, R.F., ND. 1997. *Traditional foods are your best medicine: improving health and longevity with native nutrition.* (Originally published in 1987 under title: *Native Nutrition: eating according to ancestral wisdom*) Rochester, Vermont: Healing Arts Press. (Originally published 1987, 1994.)

Schwarzbein, D., MD, and N. Deville. 1999. *The Schwarzbein principle.* Deerfield Beach, FL: Health Communications, Inc.

Stanford, C.B. 1999. *The hunting apes: meat eating and the origins of human behavior.* New Jersey: Princeton University Press.

Stefansson, V. 1956. Foreward of *The fat of the land* by P.D. White, MD. The Macmillan Company, enlarged edition of *Not by bread alone,* 1946.

Stefansson, V. 1922. *Hunters of the great north.* New York: Harcourt, Brace and Company.

Articles:

Abrams, H.L., Jr. 1987. "The preference for animal protein and fat: a cross cultural survey," *Food and evolution: toward a theory of human food habits,* Marvin Harris and Eric Ross, eds., Temple University Press, PA.

Bogin, Barry. "The evolution of human nutrition" *The Anthropology of Medicine.*

Bryant, V.M., Jr., and G. Williams-Dean. "The coprolites of man" *Scientific American.* January 1975.

Byrnes, S., ND, RNCP, "High protein diets: separating fact from fiction," *Power Health,* www.powerhealth.net/protein2001.htm

———. 2000. "The myth of vegetarianism" *Townsend Letter,* (July), Issue #204.

Carper, J. 1998. "Modern Stone Age food: your body craves nutrients caveman ate" *USA Weekend,* Archive, May 1–3.

Challem, J. "Paleolithic nutrition: your future is in your dietary past." *Nutrition Science News,* April, 1997.

Cordain, L., PhD, "Are higher protein intakes responsible for excessive calcium excretion?" www.beyondveg.com

———. "Dietary macronutrient ratios and their effect on biochemical indicators of risk of heart disease: comparing high-protein/low-carbohydrate diets vs. high-carbohydrate/low-fat diets." www.beyondveg.com

———. 2002. "Metabolic evidence of human adaptation to increased carnivory," and "Cave men diets offer insights to today's health problems," *Mercola Newsletter,* Feb. 23.

———.1998. interviewed by R. Crayhon, MS. "The Paleolithic diet and its modern implications." *Townsend Letter,* November, issue #184.

Day, C, 2000. "Strict vegan diets may be dangerous, especially for expectant mothers and children." *Chet Day's Health and Beyond Weekly Newsletter,* July 14.

Dye, D. "Calorie restriction may help reduce the risk of carcinoma" *Life Extension Foundation Web site: http://search.lef.org/cgi-src-bin/MsmGo. exe?grab_id=0&page_id=1312&query=mTOR&hiword=mTOR%20*

Eaton, S.B., MD, and S.B. Eaton III. "Evolution, diet and health." Atlanta, GA: Emory University, Departments of Anthropology and Radiology.

Fallon, S. and M. Enig, PhD. 1999. "Caveman cuisine." *Price-Pottenger Nutrition Foundation Health Journal,* vol. 21, No. 2.

Hirschorn, A. "Evolutionary nutrition."

Isaac, G., "The Diet of Early Man" *World Archaeology,* February 1971.

Larsen, C.S. 2000. "Reading the bones of La Florida: new approaches are offering insight into the lives of Native Americans after the Europeans arrived. Their health declined, not only because of disease but because of their altered diet and living circumstances." *Scientific American,* June, 2000: 80–85

Lewin, R., 1997. "Ancestral echoes: were the forebears of today's Europeans ancient hunter-gatherers or late arrivals armed with agricultural know-how? New genetic research suggests that Europeans may be less modern than they think." *New Scientist,* July 5, 1997.

Lindeberg, S. "On the benefits of ancient diets." http://www.Paleodiet.com

Mercola, J. MD, 2002. "The naïve vegetarian, part I." *Mercola Newsletter.* 2/2/02.

———"The naïve vegetarian, part II." *Mercola Newsletter.* 2/9/02.

———"The naïve vegetarian, part III." *Mercola Newsletter.* 2/13/02.

———"The naïve vegetarian, part IV." *Mercola Newsletter.* 2/16/02.

Auditory: Interview with Ron Rosedale, 2008

News-Medical.Net, 2004. "Investigation into mTOR protein function is far from over." referenced on: 12 Aug, 2004. at http://wi.mit.edu

Nicholson, W. 1998. interview on "Palelothic diet vs. vegetarianism: what was humanity's original, natural diet?" http://www.beyondveg.com/ nicholson.w/hb/hbinterview1a.shtml#top

——— 1999. "Longevity and health in ancient Paleolithic vs. Neolithic peoples: not what you have been told." 1997, 1999. http://www.beyondveg. com/billings-t/comp-anat-9d.shtml

——— "Rationalizations in response to the evolutionary and hunter-gatherer evidence for omnivorous diets." http://www.beyondveg.com/billings-t/ comp.anat/comp-anat-9d.shtml

Stefansson, V. 1935. "Adventures in diet, part I." *Harper's Monthly Magazine,* December 1935: 668–75.

———— "Adventures in diet, part II." *Harper's Monthly Magazine.* January, 1936: 46–54.

———— "Adventures in diet, part III." *Harper's Monthly Magazine.* February, 1936: 178–89.

Withers, M.L. 2003. "Researchers Find New Piece of Cell Growth Puzzle" *Molecular Cell,* April 9 Vol. 11, issue 4.

Technical:

Abraham, R.T. and J.J. Gibbons. 2007. "The mammalian target of Rapimycin signaling pathway: twists and turns in the road to cancer therapy." *Clin Cancer res* 13 (11): 3109–3114.

Abrams, H.L., Jr. 1980. "Vegetarianism: an anthropological/nutritional evaluation." *Journal of Applied Nutrition.* 32:2.

Aiello, L.C., et al. 1995. "The relationship of dietary quality and gut efficiency to brain size/The expensive-tissue hypothesis: the brain and the digestive System in human and primate evolution." *Current Anthropology,* April, vol. 36, no. 2: 199–221.

Asnaghi, L., et al. 2004,"MTOR: a protein kinase switching between life and death." *Pharmacol Res.* Dec; 50 (6): 545–549.

Blum, M., MD, et al. 1989 "Protein intake and kidney function in humans: its effect on 'normal aging'." *Arch Intern Med,* January, vol. 149.

Bower, B. 1987. "The 2-million-year-old meat and marrow diet resurfaces." *Science News.* January 3: 7

Cordain, L., PhD, et al. 2000. "Plant-animal subsistence ratios and macronutrient energy estimations in worldwide hunter-gatherer diets." *American Journal Clinical Nurition.* Mar,1(3): 682–92.

De, A.K. 1983. "Some biochemical parameters of aging in relation to dietary protein." *Mechanisms of Aging and Development.* Vol. 21, 37–48.

Deldicque, L, et al. 2005. "Regulation of mTOR by amino acids and resistance exercise in skeletal muscle." *European Journal Applied Physiology.* 94 (1–2): 1–10.

Eaton, M.D., S. Boyd, et al. 1997. "Paleolithic nutrition revisited: a twelve-year retrospective on its nature and implications." *European Journal of Clinical Nutrition.* 207–216.

Easton, et al. 2006 "MTOR and cancer therapy." *Oncogene* 25 (48): 6436–6446.

Gannon, M.C. "Effect of protein ingestion on the glucose appearance rate in people with type 2 diabetes." *The Journal of Clinical Endocrinology and Metabolism,* Vol. 86, Iss. 3, 1040–1047.

Inoki, K., et al., 2005. "Dysregulation of the TSC-mTOR pathway in human disease." *Nature Genetics,* 37: 19–24.

Jia, K., et al. 2004. "The TOR pathway interacts with the insulin signaling pathway to regulate C. elegans larval development, metabolism and life span." *Development* 131, 3897–3906.

Kapahi, P., et al. 2004. "Regulation of lifespan in Drosophila by modulation of genes in the mTOR signaling pathway." *Current Biology* 14, 885–890.

Kerstetter, J.E., et al. 1998. "Dietary Protein Affects Intestinal Calcium Absorption." *American Journal Clinical Nutrition,* 68: 859–65.

Lariviere, F. 1994. "Effect of dietary protein restriction on glucose and insulin metabolism in normal and diabetic humans." *Metabolism,* Vol. 43, Iss.4: 462–467.

Leopold, A.C., and R. Ardrey. 1972. "Toxic substances in plants and the food habits of early man" *Science,* May 5.

Lieb, C.W. 1926. "The effects of an exclusive long-continued meat diet, based on the history, experience and clinical survey of Vilhjalmur Stefansson, Arctic Explorer." *JAMA,* July 3.

———. 1929. "The effects on human beings of a twelve-months' exclusive meat diet." *JAMA,* July 6.

MacLennan, A. 2001. "Women's risk of intraparenchymal hemmorrhage linked to low meat and saturated fat intake." *Circulation,* 103: 856.

Powers, R.W., III, et al., 2006. "Extension of chronological life span in yeast by decreased TOR pathway signaling." *Genes Development* 20, 174–184.

Receveur, O., et al. 1996. "Variance in food use in Dene/Metis communities." *CINE Report,* October, 1996.

———. 1998. "Yukon first nations assessment of dietary benefit:risk." *CINE Report,* May, 1998.

Simopoulos, A.P. (ed.). 1999. "Evolutionary aspects of nutrition and health: diet, exercise and chronic disease." *World Review of Nutrition and Dietetics,* Washington, D.C.: Vol. 84.

Spencer, H. 1998. "Do protein and phospholipids cause calcium loss?" *Journal of Nutrition.* 118: 657–660.

Stahl, A.B. 1984. "Hominid dietary selection before fire." *Current Anthropology,* April, vol. 25, no. 2: 151–68.

Tokunaga, C., et al. 2004. "MTor integrates amino acid- and energy-sensing pathways." *Biochem Biophys Res Commun.* 313 (2): 443–446.

Wheat, J.B. 1972. "The Olsen-Chubbuck site: a paleo-Indian bison kill." *American Antiquity,* January, vol. 37, no. 1, part 2. (*Memoir of the Society of American Archaeology,* Number 26).

Wullschleger, S., et al. 2006. "MTOR signaling in growth and metabolism." *Cell* 124 (3): 471–84.

Wolfe, B.M. 1995. "Potential role of raising dietary protein intake for reducing risk of atherosclerosis." *Canadian Journal of Cardiology,* Oct., vol. 11, suppl. G.

Grains/Carbohydrates/Insulin

Books and Medical Journals:

Allan, C.B. and W. Lutz, MD. 2000. *Life without bread: excess carbohydrates as the underlying cause of disease.* Los Angeles: Keats Publishing.

Braly, J., MD, and R. Hoggan, MA, 2002. *Dangerous Grains.* New York, NY: Penguin Putnam, Inc.

Case, S. 2006. *Gluten-Free Diet.* Regina, Saskatchewan, Canada: Case nutrition consulting, originally printed in 2001.

Cohen, M.N 1989. *Health and the Rise of Civilization.* New Haven, CT: Yale University Press.

Dekker, J.M., C. Girman, et al. 2005. "Metabolic syndrome and 10-year cardio-vascular disease risk in the Hoorn study." *Circulation.* Aug 2; 112(5): 666–73.

Haffner, S.M. 2006. "Risk constellations in patients with the metabolic syndrome: epidemiology, diagnosis, and treatment patterns." *American Journal Medicine.* May; 119(5), Suppl. 1: S3–9.

Lakka, H.M., et al. 2002. "The metabolic syndrome and total and cardiovascular disease mortality in middle-aged men." *JAMA.* Dec 4; 288 (21): 2709–16.

Lieberman, S., PhD, CNS, FACN. 2007. *The gluten connection: how gluten sensitivity may be sabotaging your health.* New York, NY: Rodale Books.

Manrique, C., et al. 2005. "Hypertension and the cardiometabolic syndrome." *Journal Clinical Hypertension* Aug; 7(8): 471–6.

Messier, C. and K. Teutenberg. 2005. "The role of insulin, insulin growth factor, and insulin-degrading enzyme in brain aging and Alzheimer's disease." *Neural Plast.* 12(4): 311–28.

Peskin, B.S., professor emeritus. 2001. *Peak performance—radiant health: moving beyond the zone.* Houston, TX: Noble Publishing.

Reaven, G., MD, T.K. Strom, MBA, and B. Fox, PhD. 2000. *Syndrome X.* New York: Simon and Schuster.

Simontacchi, C. 2000. *The Crazy Makers.* New York: Mast Tarcher/Putnam Books.

Articles:

Brasco, J., MD, "Low Carbohydrate Diets." *Mercola Newsletter.*

———— "Low grain and carbohydrate diets treat hypoglycemia, heart disease, diabetes, cancer and nearly all chronic illness." *Mercola Newsletter.*

Cerami, A., H. Vlasara, and M. Brownlee. 1987. "Glucose and aging" *Scientific American.* May, 90–96.

Coleman, J. "Opioids in common food products." (working article)

Cordain, L., PhD, "The late role of grains and legumes in the human diet, and biochemical evidence of their evolutionary discordance." www. beyondveg.com

Fox, D. 2000. "Cut the carbs." *New Scientist,* March 18.

Petersen, K.F. and G.I. Shulman. 2006. "Etiology of insulin resistance." American Journal of Medicine. May; 119(5) Suppl. 1: S10–6

Rosedale, R., MD, "Diabetes is not a disease of blood sugar!" http://life-enthusiast.com/index/Articles/Rosedale/Diabetes_Is_Not_a_Disease_ Of_Blood_Sugar

————. 1999. "Insulin and its metabolic effects." presented at *Designs for Health Institute's BoulderFest* August seminar.

Saks, B.S. and D.C., Brett, "The adverse effects of wheat and other grains." *www.Paleodiet.com*

Stobbe, M. 2008. "Study: Low-carb diet best for weight, cholesterol." Medical writer for *Associated Press* July 17, 12:27 AM EDT.

Stoll, W., MD, 1998. "Sugar and immunty: leukocytic index proves the devastating effect of refined carbohydrates on immunity." www.paleodiet.com

Technical:

Abrams, H.L., 1975. "Sugar—a cultural complex and its impact on modern society." *Journal of Applied Nutrition,* Fall: 27:2.

Calle E.E. and R. Kaaks. 2004. "Overweight, obesity and cancer: epidemiological evidence and proposed mechanisms." *Nat Rev Cancer.* Aug., 4(8): 579–91.

Capeau J. 2005., "Insulin signaling: mechanisms altered in insulin resistance." *Med Sci (Paris).* Dec. 21 Spec. No: 34–9.

Cordain, L., PhD, 1999. "Cereal grains: humanity's double-edged sword." *World Review of Nutrition and Dietetics,* vol. 84: 19–73.

Fields, M. 1984. *Proceedings of the Society of Experimental Biology and Medicine,* 175: 530–537.

Foster, et al. 2003. "A randomized trial of a low-carbohydrate diet for obesity. *New England Journal of Medicine,* 348 (21): 2082–2090.

Freed, D.J. 1999. "Do dietary lectins cause disease?" editorial appearing in *BMJ* 17 April, 318: 1023–1024.

Ginsberg, Henry, et al., 1976. "Induction of Hypertriglyceridemia by a low-fat diet." from the Dept. of Medicine, Stanford University School of Medicine and Veterans Administration Hospital, Palo Alto, CA. *Journal Clinical Endocrinology Metabolism,* 42: 729.

Halton et al. 2006. "Low-carbohydrate-diet score and the risk of coronary heart disease in women. *New England Journal of Medicine.* 355 (19): 1991–2002.

Heller, R.F. and Rachael F. Heller. 1994. "Hyperinsulinemic obesity and carbohydrate addiction: the missing link is the carbohydrate frequency factor." *Medical Hypotheses.* 42: 307–312.

———. 1996. "Intake of Macronutrients and Risk of Breast Cancer." *The Lancet,* Vol. 349, May 18.

Ho, et al. 2007. "AGFD 232—Food bioactives and neutraceuticals: production, chemistry, analysis and health effects." Paper regarding biological effects of high fructose corn syrup presented at symposium of *American Chemical Society,* Boston, MA: August 23.

Jeppsen, J., et al. 1997. "Effect of low-fat, high carbohydrate diets on risk factors for Ischemic heart disease in post menopausal women." *American Journal Clinical Nutrition.* 65: 1027–33.

Reaven, G.M. 1995. "Pathophysiology of insulin resistance in human disease." *Physiological Reviews,* July, vol. 75, No. 3.

Wadley, G., at al. 1993. "The origins of agriculture—a biological perspective and a new hypothesis." *Australian Biologist.* June, 6: 96–105.

Yudkin, J., MA, MD, PhD, 1971. "Sugar consumption and myocardial infarction" *Lancet* 1:296–297.

———. 1969. "Sucrose and heart disease." *Lancet,* 14:16–20.

———. 1967. "Sugar intake and myocardial infarction." *American Journal Clinical Nutrition,* 20: 503.

———. 1964. "Levels of dietary sucrose in patients with occlusive atherosclerotic disease." *Lancet.* July 4.

———. 1964. "Dietary fat and dietary sugar in relation to Ischemic heart disease and diabetes" *Lancet.* 2, 4.

Soy

Books:

Daniel, K.T. 2005. *The whole soy story: the dark side of America's favorite health food.*

———. 2005. Interview, "Facts about soy the industry doesn't want you to know." PDF download on April 12, 2008.

Fallon, S. and M. Enig. 1999. *Nourishing traditions: the cookbook that challenges politically correct nutrition and the diet dictocrats.* ProMotion Publishing.

Articles:

———. 1997. "Monsanto genetically engineered soya has elevated hormone levels: public health threat." October, 1997: http://www.holisticmed.com/

———. "Toxicity from genetically-engineered foods." http://www.holisticmed.com/

———. "Soy supplements fail to help menopausal symptoms." *Mercola Newsletter.*

———. "Link between high soy diet during pregnancy and nursing and eventual developmental changes in children." *Mercola Newsletter.*

———. 2000. "Scientists protest FDAs soy protein ruling." *Nexus Magazine,* November-December: 11–13.

———. "Concerns regarding soybeans." http://www.rheumatic.org/soy.htm

Altonn, H. 1999. "Too much tofu induces 'brain aging,' study shows." *Honolulu Star Bulletin,* Friday, November 19, 1999.

Fallon, S. and M. Enig, PhD. 2000. "Tragedy and hype: the third international soy symposium." *Nexus Magazine,* April–May: 17–22/73–74.

———. "The Ploy of Soy." *Weston A. Price Foundation Web site:* www.WestonAPrice.org

———. 1995. "Concerns Regarding Soybeans." *Health Freedom News,* September.

Finucan, B. and C. Gerson. 2000. "Soy: too good to be true, Parts 1 & 2." *Mercola Newsletter,* issue # 140 & 141, February 13 & 20, 2000.

Fitzpatrick, M., PhD, MNZIC, "Soy isoflavones: panacea or poison?" *Weston A. Price Foundation Web site:* www.WestonAPrice.org

Goddard, I.W. "Is there reason to believe tofu may cause brain atrophy?" http://www.soyonlineservice.co.nz

———. 1997. "Soybean products: a recipe for disaster?" *Nexus Magazine,* April–May, Vol. 4, No. 3.

Hanson, M., PhD and J. Halloran, "Jeapordizing the future? Genetic engineering, food and the environment." *Consumer Policy Institute/Consumers Union:* http://www.pmac.net/

Liebovitz, B., PhD, 1995. "Soy protein: sorting out the science." *Muscular Development, Fitness and Health.* December.

MacArthur, J.D. 2000. "The trouble with tofu: soy and the brain." *Mercola Newsletter,* September 17, issue # 171.

Schardt, David. 2000. "Phytoestrogens for menopause." *Nutrition Action Newsletter.* Jan/Feb: Center for Science in the Public Interest—U.S. Edition.

Sheehan, D.M., PhD, director, Estrogen Base Program, Division of Genetic and Reproductive Toxicology, and Doerge, D.R., PhD, Division of Biochemical Toxicology. Letter written to FDA regarding opposition to health claims for soy products fully referenced. Found online at www.soyonlineservice.co.nz

Technical:

1999. "Soy Can Cause Severe Allergic Reactions." *Allergy.* 54: 261–265.

Ardies, C.M. et al., 1998. "Xenoestrogens significantly enhance risk for breast cancer during growth and adolescence." *Medical Hypotheses,* June 50: 6 457–64.

Atluru, S. and D. Atluru. 1991. "Evidence that genestein, a protein-tyrosine kinase inhibitor, inhibits CD28 monoclonal antibody-stimulated human T-cell proliferation." *Transplantation.* Feb 51: 2, 448–50.

Canaris, G.J., MD, MSPH, et al. 2000. "The Colorado thyroid disease prevalence study." *Arch Intern Med.* 160: 526–534.

Connolly, J.M., et al. 1997. "Effects of dietary Manhadan oil, soy and a cyclooxygenase inhibitor on human breast cancer cell growth and metastesis in nude mice." *Nutrition and Cancer.* 29 (1), 48–54.

Dees, C., et al. 1997. "Dietary estrogens stimulate human breast cells to enter the cell cycle." *Environ Health Perspect.* April 5, Suppl 3: 633–6.

Divi, R.L., et al. 1997. "Anti-thyroid isoflavones from soybean: isolation, characterization, and mechanisms of action." *Biochemical Pharmacology.* Nov 15. 54:10, 1087–96.

———., et al. 1996. "Inhibition of thyroid peroxidase by dietary flavonoids." *Chem Res Toxicol.* Jan–Feb; 9 (1): 16–23.

Fitzpatrick, M., MD, 2006. as quoted in "Should we worry about soya in our food?" by F. Lawrence, *The Guardian,* July 25, 2006.

Hsieh, C., et al. 1998. "Estrogenic effects of genistein on the growth of estrogen receptor-positive human breast cancer (MCF-7) cells in vitro and in vivo." *Cancer Research.* September 1, 58: 17, 3833–8.

Irvine, C.H., et al. 1998. "Phytoestrogens in soy-based infant foods: concentration, daily intake, and possible biological effects." *Proc Soc Exp Biol Med.* Mar. 217:3, 247–53.

Ishizuki, Y., et al. 1991. "The effects on the thyroid gland of soybeans administered experimentally in healthy subjects." *Nippon Naibunpi Gakkai Zasshi.* (Japanese) May 20. 67:5, 622–9.

Kaayla, D. 2006. as quoted in "Too much of a good thing? Controversy rages over the world's most regaled legume," by J. Nestor. *SFGate.com*, August 13, 2006.

McMichael-Phillips, D.F., et al., 1998. "Effects of soy protein supplementation on epithelial proliferation in the histologically normal human breast." *American Journal Clinical Nutrition.* Dec. 68:6. Suppl. 1431S–1435S.

Metzler, M., et al. 1998. "Genotoxicity of estrogens." *Z Lebensm Unters Forsch A.* 206: 367–73.

Morris, S.M. 1998. "P53, mutations and apoptosis in genistein-exposed human lympho blastoid cells." *Mutat Res.* Aug 31. 405:1 41–56.

2000. "Soy formulas and the effects of isoflavones on the thyroid." *New Zealand Medical Journal.* Feb 11. Volume 113.

1999. "Pregnant women should not eat soy products." *Oncol Rep.* Sept–Oct; 6 (5): 1089–95.

Petrakis, N.L., et al. 1996. "Stimulatory influence of soy protein isolate on breast secretion in pre- and post-menopausal women." *Cancer Epidemiol Biomarkers Prev.* Oct 5:10, 785–94.

Rackis J., et al. 1985. "The USDA trypsin inhibitor study, background, objectives and procedural details." *Qualification of Plant Foods in Human Nutrition.*, vol. 35.

Sacks F.M., and A. Lichtenstein, et al. 2006. "Soy protein, isoflavones, and cardiovascular health. An American Heart Association science advisory for professionals." from the Nutrition Committee. *Circulation.* 113:1034.

Setchell, K.D., et al. 1997. "Exposure of infants to phyto-oestrogens from soy-based infant formula." *Lancet.* Jul 5, 350:9070, 23–7.

Wang, C., et al. 1997. "Phytoestrogen concentration determines effects on DNA synthesis in human breast cancer cells." *Nutrition and Cancer.* 28 (3), 236–247.

White, L., et al. 1996. "Association of mid-life consumption of tofu with late

life cognitive impairment and dementia: the Honolulu-Asia aging study."
Fifth International Conference on Alzheimer's Disease, #487, 27 July 1996,
Osaka, Japan.

Dietary Fat/Heart Disease ... Etc.

(Note: many titles in the Paleolithic Diet/Protein category cover this
subject, as well)

Books:

Enig, M., PhD. 2000. *Know your fats: the complete primer for understanding
the nutrition of fats, oils and cholesterol.* Bethesda Press, April.

Enig, M., PhD, and S. Fallon. 2005. *Eat fat lose fat.* Hudson Street Press.

Erdmann, R., PhD, and M. Jones. 1995. *Fats that can save your life: the critical
role of fats and oils in health and disease.* Thorsons Publishing Limited,
1990.

Erasmus, U. 1993. *Fats that heal, fats that kill.* Burnaby, B.C., Canada: Alive
Books, 1986.

Frankel, P.,PhD, and C. Kim. 1996. Preface of *Beyond antioxidants:
methylation, homocysteine and nutrition* by C. Cooney, PhD, Researcher at
NCTR: Division of Nutritional Toxicology. The Research Corner, 1996.

Koga, Y. et al. 1994. *Recent trends in cardiovascular disease and risk factors in the
seven countries.* Study: Japan. Lessons for science from the Seven Countries
Study, Toshima, et al., eds. New York, NY: Springer. 1994, 63–74.

Mann, G.V., ed. 1993. *Coronary heart disease: the dietary sense and nonsense.*
Paul and Company Publishers. July.

Murray, M., ND, and J., Beutler, RRT, RCP. 1996. *Understanding fats and
oils: your guide to healing with essential fatty acids.* Progressive Health
Publishing.

Peskin, B.S., professor emeritus. 2001. *Peak performance—radiant health:
moving beyond the zone* Houston, TX: Noble Publishing.

Pollan, M. 2006. *The omnivore's dilemma: a natural history of four meals.* The
Penguin Press, New York.

Ravnskov, U., MD, PhD. 2000. *The cholesterol myths: exposing the fallacy that
saturated fat and cholesterol cause heart disease.* Washington, DC: New
Trends Publishing.

Robinson, J. 2000. *Why grassfed is best!: the surprising benefits of grassfed meat,
eggs and dairy products.* Vashon Island Press.

Saynor, R., MD, and F. Ryan, MD. 1990. *The Eskimo diet: how to avoid a heart
attack.* London: Ebury Press.

Schmidt, M.A. 1997. Foreward of *Smart fats: how dietary fats and oils affect mental, physical and emotional intelligence* by J.S. Bland. Berkeley, California: Frog, Ltd.

Schwarzbein, D., MD, and N. Deville. 1999. *The Schwarzbein principle.* Deerfield Beach, FL: Health Communications, Inc.

Taubes, G. 2007. *Good calories, bad calories: challenging the conventional wisdom on diet, weight control and disease.* New York, NY: Alfred A. Knopf.

Articles:

Ainsworth, C. "Love That Fat," *New Scientist,* Vol. 167, Ass .2256: 36.

American Heart Association. 2001. "Fatty fish cuts risk of death from heart attack in elderly." *Health News.* March 1.

Associated Press. 2007. "Cholesterol drug use rising rapidly in young: Experts cite higher rates of obesity, increased preventive treatments." October 30.

Byrnes, S., ND, RNCP. "Why butter is better." *Mercola Newsletter.*

Bulkeley, W.M. 2008. "Study fuels low-fat vs. low-carb debate." *The Wall Street Journal.* July 17, D1.

Conner, W. PhD. 2002. "Importance of omega three fats in health and disease." *Mercola Newsletter.* March 13.

Enig, M., PhD. "Diet, serum cholesterol, and coronary heart disease." from chapter 3: *Coronary Heart Disease: the dietary sense and nonsense.*

Enig., M., PhD. 2000. Interview: "Health Risks of Processed Foods and the Dangers of Trans Fats" by Passwater, R.A., PhD, *Mercola Newsletter.* # 157. June 10.

Fallon, S. and M. Enig, PhD, 1999. "The oiling of America." *Nexus Magazine.* Vol. 6, Number 1. December1998–January 1999.

Finn, C. 2002. "Why high carbohydrate diets are not the best way to lose weight." *Christian Finn's facts about Fitness.* February 4. www. thefactsaboutfitness.com/articles/fatloss.htm.

Mann, G.V. "A short history of the diet/heart hypothesis." from chapter 1 of: *Coronary heart disease: the dietary sense and nonsense.*

Mercola Newsletter, The. 2001. "Cholesterol is needed to help your brain cells communicate." November 24. www.mercola.com/2001/nov/24/cholesterol.htm Originally appeared in *Science,* November 9, 2001. 294:1354–1357.

Mercola Newsletter, The. 2000. "Lipoprotein(a) increases heart disease risk." September 17. www.mercola.com/2000/sept/17/lipoprotein_a.htm Originally appeared in *Circulation,* September 5, 2000:102.

Mercola, J., MD. 2002. "Breakthrough updates you need to know on vitamin D." *Mercola Newsletter.* Feb. 23.

Moore, T.J. 1989. "The Cholesterol Myth." *The Atlantic,* Vol. V264, ISS: #3, Sept. 37 (25) ISSN: 0276-9077, ATMOA.

O'Neill, M. 1991. "Can foi gras aid the heart? A french scientist says 'yes.'" *New York Times.* Nov 17.

Peat, R., PhD. "Coconut oil." *Mercola Newsletter* #205.

Raloff, J. 1996. "High fat diets help athletes perform." *Science News,* vol. 149, no. 18. May 4: 287.

Taubs, G. 2001. "The soft science of dietary fat." *Science.* March 30: Vol. 291.

———. 2002. "What if fat doesn't make you fat?" *The New York Times Magazine.* July 7.

Technical:

Alawi A, et al. 2007. "Effect of the magnitude of lipid lowering on cancer." *Journal of the American College of Cardiology,* 50 (2007): 409–418.

Aschario, A. and W.C. Willett. 1997. "Health effects of trans-fatty acids." *American Journal Clinical Nutrition.* 66 (suppl): 1006S–10S.

Beane-Rogers, J., CM, PhD, FRSC. 1995. "Are saturated fatty acids essential in the diet?" Letter to the Editor. *Nutrition Reviews.* Sept. Vol. 53, No. 9: 269.

Broadhurst, C.L. 1997. "Balanced intakes of natural triglycerides for optimum nutrition: an evolutionary and phytochemical perspective." *Medical Hypotheses.* 49, 247–261.

Carrol, K.K. and H.T. Khan. 1971 "Lipids." 6:415.

Dhingra R., et al. 2007. "Soft drink consumption and risk of developing cardiometabolic risk factors and the metabolic syndrome in middle-aged adults in the community." *Circulation.* 116: 480–488.

Dhiman, T., PhD. 1998. "Detailed fatty acid composition report of organic pasture-fed beef from River Run Farm in Clatskanie, OR." Research done at Skaggs Nutrition Laboratory, Utah State University, UT reported: October 10.

Elias, P.K., et al. 2005. "Serum cholesterol and cognitive performance in the Framingham Heart Study," *Psychosomatic Medicine.* 67(1): 24–30.

Felton, C.V., et al. 1994. "Dietary polyunsaturated fatty acids and composition of human aortic plaques." *Lancet.* 344: 1195.

Folkers, et al. 1990. "Lovastatin decreases coenzyme Q levels in humans." *Proceedings of the National Academy of Sciences.* 87(22): 8931–4.

Garrett, H.E., MD, and E.C. Horning, PhD, et al. 1964. "Serum cholesterol values in patients treated surgically for atherosclerosis." *JAMA,* August 31, vol. 189, No. 9: 655–59.

Gillman, M.W., MD, et al. 1997. "Inverse association of dietary fat with development of ischemic stroke in men." *JAMA,* December 24/31—Vol. 278, No. 24.

Golomb, B.A. 2005. "Impact of statin adverse events in the elderly." *Expert Opinion on Drug Safety.* 4(3):389–397.

Kabera, J.J. 1978. "The pharmacological effects of lipids." *The American Oil Chemists Society.* Champain, IL: 1–14.

Knopp, et al. 2004. "Saturated fats prevent coronary artery disease? An American paradox." *American Journal of Clinical Nutrition.* 80(5): 1102–1103.

Lourdes, Ribas, et al. 1995. "How could changes in diet explain changes in coronary heart disease mortality in Spain? The Spanish paradox." *American Journal of Clinical Nutrition.* 61 Suppl.: 1351S–9S.

Lutsey, P., L. Steffen, and J. Stevens. 2008. "Dietary intake and the development of the metabolic syndrome:the atherosclerosis risk in communities study." *Circulation.* 117: 754–761.

MacLennan, A. 2001 "Women's risk of intraparenchymal hemmorhage linked to low meat and saturated fat intake." *Circulation.* 103: 856.

Malhotra, S. 1968. *Indian Journal of Industrial Medicine.* 14: 219.

Mann, G., MD, et al. 1994. "Metabolic consequences of dietary trans fatty acids." *Lancet,* 343: 1268–1271.

Newbold, H.L. "Reducing serum cholesterol with a diet high in animal fat." *South Med J.* Jan; 81 (1): 61–3.

Okuyama, Harumi, et al. 1997. "Dietary fatty acids: the N-6/N-3 balance and chronic elderly diseases. Excess linoleic acid and relative N-3 deficiency syndrome seen in Japan." *Prog Lipid Res.* Vol. 35, No. 4: 409–457.

Oliver, M.F. 1997. "It is more important to increase the intake of saturated fats than to decrease the intake of saturated fats: evidence from clinical trials relating to ischemic heart disease." *American Journal of Clinical Nutrition.* 66 Suppl.: 980S–6S.

Olsen, R.E. 1998. "Evolution of ideas about the nutritional value of dietary fat." *Journal of Nutrition.* 128: 421S.

Pan, D.A. A.J. Hubert, and L.H. Storliem. 1994. "Critical review: dietary fats, membrane phospholipids and obesity." Department of Medicine, Endocrinology, University of Sydney, Australia, and Department of

Biological Sciences, University of Wollongong, Wollongong, Australia. *American Institute of Nutrition.*

Ravnskov, U. 1998. "The questionable role of saturated and polyunsaturated fatty acids in cardiovascular disease." *Journal of Clinical Epidemiology.* Vol. 51, No. 6: 443–460.

————. 1988. "Re: Golomb's dissent." *Journal of Clinical Epidemiology.* Vol. 51, No. 6: 465.

Rodney A.H., MD, T.P. Hofer, MD, MSc, and S. Vijan, MD, MSc. 2006. "Narrative review: lack of evidence for recommended low-density lipoprotein treatment targets: a solvable problem."*Annals of Internal Medicine.* 3 October, Volume 145, Issue 7: 520–530.

Salmond, C., MSc. 1981. "Cholesterol, coconuts and diet on Polynesian Atolls: a natural experiment: the Pukapuka and Tokelau Island studies." *The American Journal of Clinical Nutrition.* August. 34:1552–1561.

Shai, I., RD, PhD, and D. Schwarzfuchs, et al., 2008. "Weight loss with a low-carbohydrate, mediterranean, or low-fat diet." for the Dietary Intervention Randomized Controlled Trial (DIRECT) Group, *The New England Journal of Medicine.* July 17th. Number 3, Volume 359: 229–241.

Tavani, A., et al. 1997. "Margarine intake and risk of nonfatal acute myocardial infarction in Italian women." *European Journal of Clinical Nutrition.* 51, 30–32.

Watkins, B.A. and M.F. Seifert. 1996. "Food Lipids and Bone Health."

Yam, D., et al. 1996. "Diet and disease—the Israeli paradox: possible dangers of a high omega-6 polyunsaturated fatty acid diet." *Isr J Med Sci.* 32: 1134–1143.

Vitamin D

Books:

Hobday, R. 1999. *The healing sun: sunlight and health in the 21st Century.* Scotland: Findhorn Press. 67.

Sears, A., MD, and J. Herring *Your best health under the sun.* Self-published available by request at: 12794 Forest Hill Blvd., Suite 16, Wellington, FL 33414 2007

Sullivan, K., CN. 2006. *Naked at noon: understanding sunlight and vitamin D.* Publication forthcoming.

Articles/information:

Byrnes, S., PhD, RNCP. "Most of us need supplemental vitamin D." http://

articles.mercola.com/sites/articles/archive/2002/02/06/vegetarianism-myths-03.aspx

Cannell, J.J., MD, executive director of The Vitamin D Council, "Vitamin D lowers inflammation." http://articles.mercola.com/sites/articles/archive/2004/02/28/vitamin-d-part-twenty.aspx

Cannell, J.J., MD, and A. Vasquez, DC, ND. "Measuring your vitamin D levels: your most important blood test?" http://articles.mercola.com/sites/articles/archive/2004/07/03/vitamin-d-levels.aspx

2007. "Vitamin D supplements may lengthen life." *Forbes Magazine.* September 10.

Giovannucci, E., MD. 2006. "Reduce your cancer risks with vitamin D." *Cancer Epidemiology Biomarkers & Prevention.* November 28.

Kotz, D. 2008. "Time in the sun: how much is needed for vitamin D?" *U.S. News and World Report.* June 23.

2007. "More evidence vitamin D prevents cancer." *Science Daily* February 8.

Stein, R. 2004. "Vitamin D deficiency is major health risk." *Washington Post.* May 21.

———. 2008. "Some seek guidelines to reflect vitamin D's benefits." *Washington Post.* Friday, July 4.

Vitamin D Council: http://www.vitamindcouncil.com/

2002. "Vitamin D decreases heart disease death risk." *42nd annual conference on cardiovascular disease and epidemiology prevention in Honolulu, Hawaii.* April 23. http://articles.mercola.com/2002/may/11/vitamin_d.htm

Technical:

Garland, et al. 2005. "Vitamin D and prevention of breast cancer: Pooled analysis," *Journal of Steroid Biochemistry and Molecular Biology.* 97(1–2):179–94.

Gorham, et al. "Optimal vitamin D status for colorectal cancer prevention: a quantitative meta-analysis," *American Journal of Preventive Medicine.* 32(3): 210–216.

Grant, W.B., et al, 2006. "The association of solar ultraviolet B (UVB) with reducing risk of cancer: multifactorial ecologic analysis of geographic variation in age-adjusted cancer mortality rates," *Anticancer Research.* 26: 2687–2700.

Giovanucci, et al. 2006. "Prospective study of predictors of vitamin D status and cancer incidence and mortality in men," *Journal of the National Cancer Institute.* 98(7):451–459.

Holick, M.F. 2004. "Vitamin D: importance in the prevention of cancers, type 1 diabetes, heart disease, and osteoporosis." *American Journal of Clinical Nutrition.* March. Vol. 79, No. 3, 362–371.

Houghton, L.A. and V. Reinhold. 2006. "The case against ergocalciferol (vitamin D2) as a vitamin supplement." *American Journal of Clinical Nutrition.* October, Vol. 84, No. 4, 694–697.

Lappe, et al. 2006. "Vitamin D status in a rural postmenopausal female population," *Journal of the American College of Nutrition.* 25(5): 395–402.

2007. "High prevalence of vitamin D insufficiency in black and white pregnant women residing in the northern United States and their neonates." *Journal of Nutrition.* 137:447–452.

Munger, K.L. and S.M. Zhang, et al. 2004. "Vitamin D intake and incidence of multiple sclerosis." *Neurology.* Jan 13;62(1):60–5.

Wilkins, C.H., MD, and Y.I. Sheline, MD, et al. 2006. "Vitamin D deficiency is associated with low mood and worse cognitive performance in older adults." *Am J Geriatr Psychiatry.* December. 14:1032–1040.

Genetic Influence

Books:

Lipton, B., PhD. 2005. *The Biology of belief.* Santa Rosa, CA: Elite Books.

Pert, C. 1997. *Molecules of emotion: the science behind mind-body medicine.* New York: Scribner.

Dawkins, R., PhD. 1976. *The selfish gene.* New York: Oxford University Press, Inc.

Articles:

Pearson, H. 2003. "Geneticists play the numbers game in vain." *Nature.* 423:576.

Silverman, P.H. 2004. "Re-thinking genetic determinism: with only 30,000 genes, what is it that makes humans human?" *The Scientist.* 32–33.

Willet, W.C. 2002. "Balancing lifestyle and genomics research for disease prevention." *Science.* 296:695–698.

Technical:

Nijout, H.F. 1990. "Metaphors and the role of genes in development." *Bioessays.* 12 (9):441–446.

Waterland, R.A. and R.L. Jirtle. 2003. "Transposable elements: targets for early nutritional effects on epigenic gene regulation." *Molecular and Cell Biology.* 23 (15):5293–5300.

Digestion

Books:

Campbell-McBride. *Gut and Psychology Syndrome. Natural Treatment for Autism, Dyspraxia, Dyslexia, ADD/ADHD, Depression and Schizophrenia.* 2004. Medinform Publishing

Lipski, E., PhD, CCN. 2005. *Digestive wellness: how to strengthen the immune system and prevent disease through healthy digestion.* Third Edition. McGraw-Hill Companies.

Nelson G.J. "Dietary fat, *trans* fatty acids, and risk of coronary heart disease." *Nutrition Reviews* 56:250-252; 1998

Wright, J., MD, and L. Lenard, PhD. 2001. *Why stomach acid is good for you: natural relief from heartburn, indigestion, reflux and GERD.* M. Evans and Company.

Technical:

Little T.J., M. Horowitz M, and C. Feinle-Bisset. 2005. Role of cholecystokinin in appetite control and body weight regulation. *Obes Rev.* Nov; 6(4):297–306.

Miscellaneous Dietary Topics

Books:

Batmanghelidj, F., MD. 1995. *Your body's many cries for water.* Global Health Solutions, Inc. 1992, 1993, 1994, Second Edition: 1995.

Brownstein, D., MD 2008. *Iodine: Why you need it. Why you can't live without it.* Medical Alternatives Press, Third Edition. 2008

2004. *Clinical nutrition: a functional approach.* Second edition. Gig Harbor, Washington: Institute For Functional Medicine.

2003. *Disease prevention and treatment.* Expanded 4th edition. Life Extension Media, 2003

Fallon, S., P. Connoly, and M. Enig, PhD. 1995. *Nourishing traditions: the cookbook that challenges politically correct nutrition and the diet dictocrats.* ProMotion Publishing.

Guyton, A.C., MD, and J.E. Hall, PhD. 1996. *Textbook of medical physiology.* Ninth edition. Philadelphia, PA: W.B. Saunders Company.

Haas, E.M., MD, with B. Levin, PhD, RD. 2006. *Staying healthy with nutrition.* Berkeley, CA: Celestial Arts.

2004. *Introduction to the human body: the essentials of Anatomy and Physiology.* Sixth edition. Biological sciences Textbooks, Inc. and Sandra Reynolds Grabowski.

Moynihan, R. and A. Cassels. 2005. *Selling sickness: how the world's biggest pharmaceutical companies are turning us all into patients.* New York, NY: Nation Books.

Passwater, R.A., PhD, and E.M. Cranton, MD. 1983. *Trace elements, hair analysis and nutrition.* New Canaan, CT.

2001. *PDR for nutritional supplements.* Thomson PDR.

Peat, R., PhD. 1997. *From PMS to menopause.* Eugene, OR: Raymond Peat.

Pfeiffer, C.C., PhD, MD, and the Publications Committee of the Brain Bio Center. 1975. *Mental and elemental nutrients: a physician's guide to nutrition and healthcare.* New Canaan, CT: Keats Publishing, Inc.

Prasad, A.N., *et al.* 1979. "Alternative epilepsy therapies: the ketogenic diet, immunoglobulins and steroids." *Epilepsia.* 37 suppl. 1: S81–S95.

Rapp, D.J., MD. 1979. *Allergies and the hyperactive child.* New York: Simon and Schuster, Inc.

———. 1991. *Is this your child?: discovering and treating unrecognized allergies in children and adults.* New York: William Morrow and Company, Ltd.

Ross, J., MA. 1999. *The diet cure.* New York, NY: Penguin Putnam Inc.

Schauss, A.G., PhD, 1981. Introduction of *Diet, crime and delinquency* by Michael Lesser, MD.

Parker House, 1980.

Simontacchi, C. 2000. *The Crazy Makers: how the food industry is destroying our brains and harming our children.* Jeremy Tarcher/Putnam Books.

Stender, S. and J. Dyerberg. 2001. *Ugeskr laeger.* 163:2349–235.

Timon, M.S. 1979. *Mineral Logic: understanding the mineral transporting system* reviewed by J.S. Bland, PhD. Benjamin/Cummings Publishing Co.

Werbach, M.R., MD. 1996. *Nutritional influences on illness: a sourcebook of clinical research.* Second edition. Tarzana, CA: Third Line Press.

Wiley, T.S. 2000. *Lights out: sleep, sugar and survival.* New York, NY: Pocket Books.

Articles
General:
Anderson, F., BS. *The Thesis of Body Mineral Balancing.* Summary of research. *http://www.traceminerals.com/thesis.html*

Ashmead, D., PhD. 1981. "What a zinc deficiency can do to you." *Bestways Magazine.* April.

Biser, S. "Don't be conned by the crusade against salt." *The Newsletter of Advanced Natural Therapies.* Vol. 2, No. 6.

Block, M.A., DO. 1997. "Treating Attention Deficit Disorder naturally." *Nature's Impact.* October/November.

Bushman, J., MPH, RD. 1998. "ADD: Attention Deficit Disorder: natural therapies may offer improvement without the side effects of conventional drugs." *Co-op Consumer News,* September/October.

Dean, W., MD. 2004. "DMAE: cognitive-enhancing, life extending nutrient." *Vitamin Research News.* 18:8 1–4.

Ethridge, E. 1997. "Brain food" *Energy Times.* September.

Heinerman, J., PhD. 1997. "Mineral nutrition of coastal cultures in pre-historic times." *The Source Newsletter.* March/April.

2001. "Vegetables without Vitamins." *Life Extension Magazine.* March.

Long, T.C., and J. Tajuba, et al. 2007. "Nanosize titanium dioxide stimulates reactive oxygen species in brain microglia and damages neurons in vitro." *Environmental Health Perspectives.* November. Volume 115, Number 11.

Nielsen, M.T., professor, department of biology, University of Utah. "Ions: The Body's Electrical Energy Source." *http://traceminerals.com/ions2.html*

2007. "Doctors say, raise the RDAs now." *Orthomolecular Medicine News Service,* October 30.

Osborne, S.E., "Eat right for your type hype." *Price-Pottenger Foundation Health and Healing Wisdom Journal.* Vol. 22, No. 4.

Schauss, A., PhD. 1997. "Minerals and human health: the rationale for optimal and balanced trace element levels." http://www.traceminerals.com/humanhealth.html 4-04.

———. 1997. "An analysis of colloidal mineral claims." *Health Counselor Magazine.*

Saul, S. and G. Harris. 2007. "Diabetes drug still has heart risks, doctors warn." *New York Times.*

Sahley, B.J. 2000. "Natural control of ADD and ADHD." *Vitamin Research News.* 14 (10).

Singh, et al. 2007. "Thiazolidinediones and heart failure: A teleo-analysis." *Diabetes Care.* 30:2148–2153.

———. 2007. "Rosiglitazone and cardiovascular risk." *The New England Journal of Medicine.* 30(24):2148-2153.

Stitt, B.R. 1997. "Healing the delinquent mind: a complementary approach." *Nature's Impact.* October/November.

Sult, T., MD. "Attention Deficit Hyperactivity Disorder." *Article prepared by Immuno Laboratories, Inc. relating to food-sensitivity issues and ADD/HD.*

Weise E. 2005. "Are our products our enemy?" *USA Today.* Aug 2. http://www.pbs.org/tradesecrets/problem/bodyburden.html

Technical:

Adriani, W., et al. 2004. "Acetyl-l-carnitine reduces impulsive behaviour in adolescent rats." *Psychopharmacology.* Nov; 176 (3–4): 296–304.

Godfrey K. et al. 1996. "Maternal nutrition in early and late pregnancy in relation to placental and fetal growth." *British Medical Journal.* 42: 243–251.

Heini, A.F. and R.L. Weinsier. 1997. *"Divergent trends in obesity and fat intake patterns: the American paradox."* American Journal of Medicine. Mar., 102(3): 259–64.

Holman, P. 1996. "Treating the ectomorphic constitution." *Journal of Nutritional and Environmental Medicine.* 6:359–370.

McConnell, H., et al. 1985. "Catecholamine metabolism in the attention deficit disorder." *Medical Hypotheses.* 17(4): 305–311.

Mitchell, A.E., et al. 2007. "Ten-year comparison on the content of flavonoids in tomatoes." *The Journal of Agriculture and Food Chemistry.* 55 (15): 6154–6159.

Tankova T., et al. 2004. "Alpha lipoic acid in the treatment of autonomic diabetic neuropathy," *Rom J Intern Med.* 42(4): 457–64.

Ulloth, J.E. and C.A. Casiano. *PMID: 12562519* PubMed. De Leon M. Department of Microbiology and Immunology, East Carolina University School of Medicine.

Wang, S. 2001. "Effects of chromium and fish oil on insulin resistance and leptin resistance in obese developing rats." *Wei Sheng Yan Jiu.* Iss. 5, 284–286.

Witte J. et al. 1997. "Diet and premenopausal bilateral breast cancer: a case control study." *Breast Cancer Research and Treatment.* 42:243–251.

2005. "Body burden—the pollution in newborns." Environmental Working Group. July 14. www.ewg.org.

Endocrine/Leptin

Books:

Richards, Byron J. Mastering Leptin: The Leptin Diet, Solving Obesity and Preventing Disease, Second Edition

Rosedale, R., MD, and C. Coleman. 2004. *The Rosedale diet.* New York: Harper Resource/HarperCollins.

Talbott, S., PhD. 2002. *The Cortisol connection: why stress makes you fat and ruins your health—and what you can do about it.* Hunter House Publishers.

Wilson, J.L., ND, DC, PhD. 2001. *Adrenal fatigue: the 21st century stress syndrome.* Smart Publications.

Articles:

Rosedale, R. MD. 2008. "Insulin, leptin, diabetes, and aging: not so strange bedfellows." *Diabetes Health 01/13.* http://www.diabeteshealth.com/read/2008/01/13/5617.html

Rosedale, R. MD 2008—Auditory interview with Dr. Joseph Mercola

Technical:

Agus, M.S. 2000. "Dietary composition and physiologic adaptations to energy restriction." *American Journal of Clinical Nutrition.* Vol. 71, Iss 4, 901–907.

Ahima, R.S. 1996. "Role of leptin in the neuroendocrine response to fasting." *Nature.* Vol. 382, 250–52.

Ainslie, D.A. 2000. "Short term, high fat diets lower circulating leptin concentrations in rats." *American Journal of Clinical Nutrition.* Vol 71, 438–442.

Baile, C.A. 2000. "Regulation of metabolism and body fat mass by leptin." *Annual Review of Nutrition.* Vol. 20, 105–127.

Blum, M., M.A. Harris, SS, et al. 2003. "Leptin, body composition and bone mineral density in premenopausal women." *Caalcif. Tissue Int.* Jul; 73(1):27–32.

Cleare, A.J. 2003. "The neuroendocrinology of chronic fatigue syndrome." *Endocr Rev.* Apr; 24(2): 236–52. Section of Neurobiology of Mood Disorders, Division of Psychological Medicine, The Institute of Psychiatry, London SE5 8AZ, United Kingdom. a.cleare@iop.kcl.ac.uk

Ducy, P. 2000. "The Osteoblast: A sophisticated fibroblast under central surveillance." *Science.* Vol 289, 1502–1504.

Figlewicz, D.P. 2003. "Adiposity signals and food reward: expanding the CNS roles of insulin and leptin." *American Journal of Physiology—Regulatory, Integrative and Comparative Physiology.* Vol. 284, R882–R892.

Harkovic, M., and M. Pavlovic, et al., Institute of Endocrinology, Diabetes and Diseases of Metabolism, Clinical Centre of Serbia, Belgrade. mzarkov@eunet.yu

Harris, R., B. 2000. "Leptin—much more than a satiety signal." *Annual Review of Nutrition.* Vol. 20, 45–75.

Hauner, H. 2005. "Secretory factors from human adipose tissue and their functional role." *Proc Nutr Soc.* May; 64(2): 163–9.

Karsenty, G. 2000. "The central regulation of bone remodeling." *Trends in Endocrinology and Metabolism.* Vol 11, Iss. 10, 437–439.

Kharrazian, Datis, D.C., D.H.Sc., September 2007 in Portland, Oregon. Course "Functional Endocrinology" sponsored by Apex Energetics and the University of Bridgeport College of Chiropractic, course #PG 952/ NCCAOM, course #ACHB 404-007.

Lafafe-Poust M.H., et al. 2003. "Glucocorticoid-induced osteoporosis: pathophysiology data and recent treatments." *Joint Bone Spine.* Mar; 70(2): 109–118.

Lang, Janet R., D.C., May 2007 in Portland, Oregon. Course "Thyroid, Adrenals and Blood Sugar" sponsored by Standard Process and Lang Integrative Health Seminars.

Roberts, et al. 2004. "Salivary cortisol response to awakening in chronic fatigue system" *Br. J. Psychiatry,* Feb; 184: 136–141.

2003. "Disorder of adrenal gland function in chronic fatigue syndrome" *Srp Arh Celok Lek.* Sep–Oct;131(9–10):370–4.

Trayhurn, P. 2005. "Endocrine and signalling role of adipose tissue: new perspectives on fat." *Acta Physiol Scand.* Aug; 184 (4): 285–93.

Wadden, T.A. 1998. "Short and long term changes in serum leptin in dieting obese women: effects of caloric restriction and weight loss." *Journal of Clinical Endocrinology and Metabolism.* Vol 83, Iss. 1, 214–218.

Wust, S, et al. 2004. "Common polymorphisms in the glucocorticoid receptor gene are associated with adrenocorticoid responses to psychosocial stresses." *J. Clin. Endocrinol Metab.* Feb; 89(2): 565–573.

Exercise

Books:

Sears, A., MD. 2006 *PACE: Rediscover your native fitness.* Wellness Research Consulting, Inc.

Tsatsouline, P. 1999. *Power to the people.* Dragon Door Publications, Inc.
http://www.scribd.com/doc/2342784/Pavel-Tsatsouline-Power-To-The-People

———. 2003. *The naked warrior.* Dragon Door Publishing.

Lee, R. 2007. *The millionaire workout.* Okenzie Publishing.

Morehouse, L.E., PhD, and L. Gross. 1977. *Maximum performance.* New York: Pocket Books.

Articles:

Lee, R. "Everything you've been told about exercise might be wrong." http://articles.mercola.com/sites/articles/archive/2006/08/08/everything-youve-been-told-about-exercise-might-be-wrong—part-iv.aspx

Mercola, J., DO, "If you aren't using this type of exercise you are missing out big time." http://v.mercola.com/blogs/public_blog/if-you-aren-t-using-this-type-of-exercise-you-are-missing-out-big-time-13930.aspx

Technical:

Deldicque, L, D. Theisen, and M. Francaux. 2005. "Regulation of mTOR by amino acids and resistance exercise in skeletal muscle." *Eur. J. Appl. Physiol.* 94 (1–2): 1–10

Talanian, J.L., and D.R. Stuart, et al. 2007. "Two weeks of high-intensity aerobic interval training increases the capacity for fat oxidation during exercise in women." *J Appl Physiol* 102: 1439–1447. First published December 14, 2006; doi:10.1152/japplphysiol.01098.2006 8750-7587/07.

Long, B.C., and R. van Stavel. 1995. "Effects of exercise training on anxiety: A meta-analysis." *Journal of Applied Sport Psychology.* 7, 167–189.

Martinsen, E.W. 1994. Physical activity and depression: clinical experience. *Acta Psychiatrica Scandinavica,* 377: 23–27.

"Impact of exercise intensity on body fatness and skeletal muscle metabolism," *Metabolism* 1994; 43(7): 814–18.

Miller, W.C., et al. 1997. "A meta-analysis of the past 25 years of weight loss research using diet, exercise, and diet plus exercise intervention." *Int J Obes Relat Metab Disord.* 21(10): 941–7.

North, T.C., P. McCullagh, and Z.V. Tran. 1990. "Effect of exercise on depression." *Exercise and Sport Science Reviews,* 18: 379–415.

O'Connor, P.J., and M.A. Youngstedt. 1995. "Influence of exercise on human sleep." *Exercise and Sport Science Reviews,* 23: 105–134.

Petruzzello, S.J. and D.M. Landers, et al. 1991. "A meta-analysis on the anxiety-reducing effects of acute and chronic exercise." *Sports Medicine.* 11(3): 143–182.

Schlicht, W. 1994. "Does physical exercise reduce anxious emotions: A meta-analysis." *Anxiety, Stress, and Coping,* 6: 275–288.

TabataI, N.K, et al. 1996. "Effects of moderate-intensity endurance and high intensity intermittent training on anaerobic capacity and VO2max." *Med Sci Sports Exerc.* 1996 Oct; 28 (10):1327–1330.

Neilan, T.G., MD, and J.L. Januzzi, MD, et al. 2006. "Myocardial injury and ventricular dysfunction related to training levels among non-elite participants in the Boston marathon." *Circulation*. 114: 2325–2333

Primal Mind: Nutrition and Mental Health

Books:

Braverman, E.R. 1997. *The healing nutrients within: facts, findings and new research on amino acids*. New Canaan, CT: Keats Publishing, Inc.

Breggin, P.R., MD. 2001. *The anti-depressant fact book*. Cambridge, MA: Perseus Publishing.

Calvin, W.H. 2002. *A brain for all seasons*. London: University of Chicago Press.

Cozolino, L. 2002. *The neuroscience of psychotherapy: building and rebuilding the human brain*. New York, NY: W.W. Norton & Company, Inc.

Kolb, B. and I.Q. Whishaw. 2001. *An introduction to brain and behavior*. Worth Publishers.

LeDoux, J. *The emotional brain*. New York, NY: Touchstone.

Pert, C., PhD. *Molecules of emotion*. New York, NY: Scribner.

Pfeiffer, C.C., PhD, MD. 1975. *Mental and elemental nutrients*. New Canaan, CT: Keats Publishing.

Ross, J., MA. 2002. *The mood cure*. Penguin Putnam Inc.

Technical:

Balestreri, R. L. Fontana and F. Astengo. 1987. "A double-blind placebo controlled evaluation of the safety and efficacy of vinpocetine in the treatment of patients with chronic vascular senile cerebral dysfunction." *J-Am-Geriatr-Soc*. May; 35(5): 425–30.

Boukje, M., et al. 2007. "Fish consumption, n–3 fatty acids, and subsequent 5-y cognitive decline in elderly men." *American Journal of Clinical Nutrition*. 85(4), 1142–1147.

Flint B.M. 2005. "Oxidative mechanisms, inflammation, and Alzheimer's disease pathogenesis." Ninth International Conference on Alzheimer's Disease. June 2005.

Helisalmi, S., et al. 2006. "Association of CYP46 intron 2 polymorphism in Finnish Alzheimer's disease." *Journal of Neurology, Neurosurgery, and Psychiatry*. 77:421–42.

Kharrazian, Datis, D.C., D.H.Sc., September 2008 in Portland, Oregon. Course "Neurotransmitters & Brain" sponsored by Apex Energetics and University of Bridgeport College of Chiropractic, course #PG 952/ NCCAOM, course #ACHB 404-009.

Kirsch, I., et al. 2008. "Initial severity and antidepressant benefits: A meta analysis of data submitted to the Food and Drug Administration." *PLOS Medicine*. February 2008/Volume 5/Issue 2/e45. www.plosmedicine.org

May, A., et al. 2007. "Plasma n–3 fatty acids and the risk of cognitive decline in older adults." *American Journal of Clinical Nutrition*. 85(4), 1103–1111.

Messier, C. and K. Teutenberg. 2005. "The role of insulin, insulin growth factor, and insulin-degrading enzyme in brain aging and Alzheimer's disease." *Neural Plast*. 12(4):311–28.

Whitmer, R., et al. 2005. "Obesity in middle age and future risk of dementia." *BMJ*, 29 April.

Wu, et al. 2004. "Dietary omega-3 fatty acids normalize BDNF levels, reduce oxidative damage, and counteract learning disability after traumatic brain injury in rats." *Journal of Neurotrauma*. 21(10):1457–67.

Pyroluria

Books:

Ross, J., MA. 2002. *The mood cure*. Penguin Putnam Inc.

Pfeiffer, C.C., PhD, MD. 1988. *Nutrition and mental illness: an orthomolecular approach to balancing body chemistry*. Healing Arts Press.

Articles:

McGinnis, W., MD. 2004. "Pyroluria: hidden cause of schizophrenia, bipolar, depression, and anxiety symptoms." Orlando, 21 May 2004. http://www.alternativementalhealth.com/articles/pyroluria.htm

Pyroluria
http://www.nutritional-healing.com.au/content/articles-content.php?heading=Pyroluria

Pyroluria
http://www.drkaslow.com/html/pyroluria.html

Technical:

Hoffer. A., MD, PhD. 1995. "The discovery of kryptopyrrole and its importance in diagnosis of biochemical imbalances in schizophrenia and in criminal behavior." *J. Orthomolecular Medicine*. 10(1):3.

Hoffer, A., M.D, PhD, et al. 1961. "The presence of unidentified substances in the urine of psychiatric patients." *J Neuropsychiatry* 2: 331–362.

Hoffer, A., MD, PhD, and H. Osmond, MD. 1963. "Malvaria: a new psychiatric disease." *Acta Psychiat Scand* 39:335–366.

Jackson, J.A., MT, ASCP, PhD, BCLD, and H.D. Riordan, MD, et al. 1997. "Urinary pyrrole in health and disease." *The Journal of Orthomolecular Medicine.* 12 (2nd Quarter): 96–8.

Pfeiffer, C., PhD, MD, and A. Sohler, PhD. 1974. "Treatment of pyroluric schizophrenia (malvaria) with large doses of pyridoxine and a dietary supplement of zinc." *J. Orthomolecular Psychiatry.* 3(4):292.

Pfeiffer, C., MD, PhD, et al. 1973. "Biochemical relationship between kryptopyrrole (mauve factor and trans-3-methyl-2-hexenoic acid schizophrenia odor)." *Res Commun Chem Pathol Pharmacol.*

Pfeiffer, C., MD, PhD, et al. 1988. "Pyroluria—zinc and B6 deficiencies." *Int Clin Nutr Rev.*

Sohler, A. PhD. 1974. "A rapid screening test for pyroluria; useful in distinguishing a schizophrenic subpopulation." *J. Orthomolecular Psychiatry.* 3(4):273.

Walsh, W.J., L.B. Glab, and M.L. Haakenson. 2004. "Reduced violent behavior following biochemical therapy." *Physiol. Behav.* 82 (5): 835–9.

Aging/Anti-Aging

Books:

Walford, R.L., MD. 1983. *Maximum Life Span.* New York: Avon Books.

Pearson, D. and S. Shaw. 1982. *Life extension: a practical and scientific approach.* New York: Warner Books, Inc.

———. *Life extension companion.* New York: Warner Books, Inc.

Weindruch R., and R.L. Walford. 1988. *The retardation of aging and disease by dietary restriction.* Springfield, IL: Charles C. Thomas.

Technical:

Apfeld, J K. 1998. "C. Cell nonautonomy of C. elegans daf-2 function in the regulation of diapause and life span." *Cell* 1998, Oct 16;95(2):199–210.

Aziz, et al, 2005. "Chemoprevention of skin cancer by grape constituent resveratrol: relevance to human disease?" *The FASEB Journal.* 19(9): 1193–95.

Bluher, M 2003. "Extended longevity in mice lacking the insulin receptor in adipose tissue," *Science.* Vol. 299, Iss. 24, 572–574.

Barrows, C.H., Jr., and G.C. Kokkman. 1978. "Diet and life extension in animal model systems." *Age* 1:131.

Carlson, A.H. and F. Hoelzel, 1946. "Apparent prolongation of the life span of rats by intermittent fasting" *J. Nutrition* 31:363.

Dorman J.B., and B. Albinder. et al. 1995. "The age-1 and daf-2 genes function in a common pathway to control the life span of Caenorhabditis elegans." *Genetics*. Dec;141(4):1399–406

Duffy, P.H. 1989. "Effect of chronic caloric restriction on physiological variables related to energy metabolism in the male Fischer 344 rat." *Mechanisms of aging and development.*, Vol. 48, Iss. 2, 117–133.

Everitt, A.V., N.J. Seedsman, and F. Jones. 1980. "The effects of hypophysectomy and continuous food restriction, begun at ages 70 and 400 days, on collagen aging, proteinuria, incidence of pathology and longevity in the male rat." *Mechanisms of aging and development.* 12:161.

Fernandez-Galaz, C. 2002. "Long term food restriction prevents aging-associated central leptin resistance in wistar rats." *Diabetologia,* 2 Vol. 45, Iss. 7, 997–1003.

Garvin, et al,. 2006. "Resveratrol induces apoptosis and inhibits angiogenesis in human breast cancer xenografts in vivo," Cancer Letters. 231(1): 113–22.

Hansen, B.C. 2001. "Symposium: Calorie restriction: Effects on body composition, insulin signaling and aging." *Journal of Nutrition,* 2001, Vol. 131, 900S-902S

Harper, et al. 2007. "Resveratrol suppresses prostate cancer progression in transgenic mice," *Journal of Carcinogenesis.* 28(9):1946–1953.

Heilbronn L.K., de JL, Frisard MI, et al. 2006. "Effect of 6-month calorie restriction on biomarkers of longevity, metabolic adaptation, and oxidative stress in overweight individuals: a randomized controlled trial." *JAMA.* Apr 5; 295(13):1539–48.

Howitz, et al. 2003. "Small molecule activators of sirtuins extend Saccharomyces cerevisiae lifespan," *Nature.* 425(6954):191–6.

Hsin, H. and C. Kenyon. 1999. "Signals from the reproductive system regulate the life span of C. elegans. development." Feb; 126(5):1055–64.

Hursting, S., D 2003. "Calorie restriction, aging and cancer prevention: mechanisms of action and applicability to humans." *Annual Review of Medicine.* Vol. 54, 131–152.

Jia, K., D. Chen, and D.L. Riddle. 2004. "The TOR pathway interacts with the insulin signaling pathway to regulate C. elegans larval development, metabolism and life span." *Development.* 131, 3897–3906.

Kalant, N. and J. Stewart., et al. 1988. "Effect of diet restriction on glucose metabolism and insulin responsiveness in aging rats." *Mech Aging Dev.* Dec; 46(1–3): 89–104.

Kapahi, P., B.M. Zid, et al. 2004. "Regulation of lifespan in Drosophila by modulation of genes in the mTOR signaling pathway." *Curr Biol* 14, 885–890.

Kealy, R.D., D.F. Lawler, et al. 2002. "Effects of diet restriction on life span and age-related changes in dogs." *J Am Vet Med Assoc.* May 1; 220(9): 1315–20.

Kenyon, C., J. Chang, et al. 1993. "A C. elegans mutant that lives twice as long as wild type." *Nature.* Dec 2; 366(6454): 461–4; comment in: *Nature.* 1993 Dec 2; 366(6454): 404–5.

Lagouge, et al. 2006. "Resveratrol improves mitochondrial function and protects against metabolic disease by activating SIRT1 and PGC-1alpha," *Cell.* 127(6): 1109–22.

Lane, M.A. and D.K. Ingram, et al. 1997. "Dehydroepiandrosterone sulfate: a biomarker of primate aging slowed by calorie restriction." *J Clin Endocrinol Metab.* Jul; 82(7): 2093–6.

Lemon, J.A., D.R. Boreham, et al. 2005. "A complex dietary supplement extends longevity of mice." *J Gerontol A Biol Sci Med Sci.* Mar; 60(3): 275–9.

Lin K., H. Hsin, et al. 2001. "C. Regulation of the Caenorhabditis elegans longevity protein DAF-16 by insulin/IGF-1 and germline signaling." *Nat Genet.* Jun; 28(2): 139–45.

Masoro, E.J. 1998. "Hormesis and the antiaging action of dietary restriction." *Exp Gerontol.* Jan–Mar; 33(1–2): 61–6.

———. "Subfield History: Caloric restriction, slowing aging, and extending life,." sageke.sciencemag.org/cgi/content/fullsageke;2003/8/re2

Masoro, E.J., B.P. Yu, et al. 1982. "Action of food restriction in delaying the aging process." *Proc Natl Acad Sci U S A.* Jul; 79(13): 4239–41.

Mattison, J.A. 2001. "Endocrine effects of dietary restriction and aging: The National Institute of Aging Study." *Journal of Anti-Aging Medicine.* Vol. 4, Iss. 3, 215–234.

Merry, B.J. 2002. "Molecular mechanisms linking calorie restriction and longevity." *Int J Biochem Cell Biol.* Nov; 34(11): 1340–54.

Nelson, D.W. 2003. "Insulin worms its way into the spotlight." *Genes and Development.* Vol. 17, 813–818.

Nicolas, A.S., D. Lanzmann-Petithory, et al. 1999. "Caloric restriction and aging." *J Nutr Health Aging.* 3(2): 77–83.

Partridge, L. "Mechanisms of Aging: public or private?" *Nature Reviews, Genetics.* Vol. 3, Iss. 3, 173.

Powers, R.W., III, M. Kaeberlein, et al. 2006. "Extension of chronological life span in yeast by decreased TOR pathway signaling." *Genes Dev* 20, 174–184.

Rae, M. 2004. "It's never too late: caloric restriction is effective in older mammals." *Rejuvenation Res.* Spring; 7(1): 3–8

Roth, G.S. 2002. "Biomarkers of caloric restriction may predict longevity in humans." *Science.* Vol. 297, Iss. 2, 811.

———. 2000. "Effects of reduced energy intake on the biology of aging: the primate model." *European Journal of Clinical Nutrition.* Vol. 54, Iss. S3, S15–S20.

Shimokawa,, I. 2001. "Leptin and anti-aging action of caloric restriction." *The Journal of Nutrition, Health and Aging.* Vol. 5, 43–48.

———. 2001. "Leptin signaling and aging: insight from caloric restriction" *Mechanisms of Aging and development.* Vol 122, Iss. 14, 1511–1519.

Sinclair, D.A. and L. Guarente. 2006. "Unlocking the secrets of longevity genes." *Scientific American.* 294 (3): 48–57.

Subbiah, M.T.R., and R.G. Siekert, Jr. 1979. "Dietary restriction and the development of Atherosclerosis." *J. Nutrition.* 41:1.

Tannenbaum, A. 1945. "The dependence of tumor formation on the composition of the calorie-restricted diet as well as on the degree of restriction." *Cancer Res.* 5: 616–25.

Wang, et al. 2007. "Effects of red wine and wine polyphenol resveratrol on platelet aggregation in vivo and in vitro." *International Journal of Molecular Medicine.* 9 (1): 77–9.

Weindruch, R.H., J.A. Kristie, et al. 1979. "The influence of controlled dietary restriction on immunologic function and aging." *Federation Proceedings.* 38: 2007.

Weindruch, R.H., S.R.S. Gottesman, and R.L. Walford. 1982. "Modification of age-related immune decline in mice dietarily restricted from or after mid-adulthood." *Proc. Nat. Acad. Sci. U.S.A.* 79: 898.

Wolkow, C.A., K.D. Kimura, et al. 2000. "Regulation of C. elegans life span by insulinlike signaling in the nervous system." *Science.* Oct 6; 290(5489): 147–50.

Yu, B.P. 1996. "Aging and oxidative stress: modulation by dietary restriction." *Free Radic Biol Med.* 21(5): 651–68.

Yu, B.P. and H.Y. Chung. 2001. "Stress resistance by caloric restriction for longevity." *Ann N Y Acad Sci.* Apr; 928:39–47.

Zern, et al. 2005. "Grape polyphenols exert a cardioprotective effect in pre- and postmenopausal women by lowering plasma lipids and reducing oxidative stress." *The Journal of Nutrition.* 135(8): 1911–7.

INDEX

Page numbers in *italics* indicate figures and tables.

blood-brain barrier, 249, 280, 282

blood sugar and glucose metabolism
    overview, 136–140
    brain function and, 242–243
    diabetes and, 152
    dietary fats and, 142
    glycemic index and, 187–189
    hormonal dysregulation and,
      148–149, 234
    onset of diabetes and, 153–154
    stress response and, 236–238

blood tests
    glucose, 138
    vitamin D and, 103–105, 314

blood thinning medication, omega-3
    supplementation and, 116

body
    mind-body connection, 231–232
    subconscious mind and, 229

body fat
    as endocrine organ, 145
    insulin and, 151
    weight loss and, 159–161

bones composition and nutrients,
    154–157

brain
    arachadonic acid and, 119
    blood-brain barrier, 249
    cholesterol and, 89
    development of, 31–32
    DHA and, 108
    diet and overall brain health, 234,
      241–246, 250–251
    EMF pollution and, 301–302
    exercise and, 285–286
    fat requirements of, 241–246
    fatty acids and, 32, 243–246
    memory and brain health
      improvement, 255–258, 273

mind-body connection, 231–232
nutritional requirements, 231, 255
serotonin and mood, 82
size of, 111
stress response and, 236–238,
    254–255, 291–295

Brain-Derived Neurotrophic Factor
    (BDNF), 286

brain-gut linkage, 82

breakfast, sample menu, 321

breast milk, 97, 123–124

breath therapy, 292

Brownstein, David, 252, 270

butter, 55, 192

butyric acid, 192

C

C. elegans, 220

cabbage juice, 77

caffeine
    Adrenal Stress Index and, 201–202
    dehydration and, 205
    elimination from diet, 178
    glucose dysregulation and, 168
    memory and, 256

caloric intake
    caloric restriction and
      antioxidants, 218
    caloric restriction and insulin
      activity, 220–222
    calorie counting and weight loss,
      163–164
    cancer and, 208–209
    complete proteins and, 207
    fatty acids and, 129
    lifespan extension and, 216–220

Campbell-McBride, Natasha, 290

cancer
    artificial sweeteners and, 186

functions and need for, 89–90, 92, 95

heart disease and, 90–94, *95*, *96*, 117

information resources, 343

molecular structure, *94*

oxidized, 54

chromium supplements, 176

chronic efforting, 276

chronic fatigue
Adrenal Stress Index and, 201–202
dehydration and, 205
loss of lean tissue and, 155
sunlight and, 281

Churchill, Winston, 310

chyme, 70, 72–73

CLA (conjugated linolenic acid), pasture-fed butter and, 55

cod liver oil, 101, 102, 114, 116, 129, 314, 329, 343

Coenzyme Q10 (CoQ10)
omega-3 fatty acids and, 114, 116
statin drugs and, 90
supplements, 177, 330

cognitive and emotional dysregulation
acetylcholine precursor supplements and, 272
brain health and, 234–235
iron deficiency and, 262–264
neurofeedback approach to treatment, 234
zinc deficiency and, 260

colloidal minerals, 259–260, 314–315

Community Supported Agriculture (CSA) programs, 52–53, 309, 313

conjugated linolenic acid (CLA)
grass-fed meat and, 84
pasture-fed butter and, 55

see also omega-3 fatty acids

cooking with fire, 31

copper, 183, 261

coprolites, 30

Cordain, Loren, 29, 342

Corn Refiners Association, 185

coronary heart disease (CHD)
cholesterol and, 90–94, *95*, *96*, 117
diet-heart hypothesis, 38
dietary fats and, 83, 86–87
incidence of, 34
trans fats and, 125
unsaturated fats and, 93–94

cortisol
chronic stress and dysglycemia, 198, 200–202, *201*, *202*, 291–292
exercise and, 171
immune system and, 79
memory and, 254
secretory IgA (SIgA) and, 162

CRON (caloric restriction with optimal nutrition), 217–218

CSA (Community Supported Agriculture) programs, 52–53

cytochrome P-448/450 and metabolism, 124

D

D-phenylalanine supplements, 284

D6D (delta-6 desaturase), 108, 111–112, 114, 117–118, 124, 127, 130

DAF-2 gene, 221

dairy products, 54–55, 81, 318, 342, 343

Danish Nutrition Council, 125

deglycyrrhizinated (DGL) licorice, 77

dehydration, 205–206

fats (*continued*)

  dietary availability and
consumption of, *35*, *36*, 175, 236

  dietary carbohydrates and, 161–162

  dietary protein and, 97, 211

  differences in structure, digestion,
and physiological effects, 87–88

  digestion optimization and, 76

  as energy source, 142, 157–158, 214

  healthy, 149

  hunter-gatherer dietary levels of,
30, 31, 34

  leptin and fat cells, 145

  longevity and, 226

  physiological purpose, 165

  see also hydrogenated oils; rancid
fats; saturated fats; unsaturated
fats; vegetable oils

fatty acids

  grain-fattened animals and, 51

  human brain and, 32

  see also essential fatty acids (EFAs)

FDA (Food and Drug Administration), 300, 301, 309

fermented foods, 67, 76–77, 81, 318

fiber, 191–193

fight or flight response

  adrenaline and, 247–248

  nervous system over-arousal and,
235

  stress management and, 293–294

fire, human use of, 31

fish oil, 113–116, 250, 256, 257, 313–314

5-HTP supplements, 272, 283

flax seed oil, 113–114, 116–117,
313–314

fluid intake, 76, 321

folic acid, 73, 250, 282, 283

food industry, 63, 306

food sensitivities

  overview, 287–290

  ADHD and, 250

  adrenal function and, 199

  cognitive and emotional
dysregulation and, 234

  elimination diets and, 288, 289,
315–316

  memory and, 254, 256

  symptoms, 287–288

  vegetarianism and, 235

foods

  conscious choices and, 311, 313

  cravings, 284, 288

  fermented, 67, 76–77, 81, 318

  high-glycemic, 247–248

  importance of chewing, 72, 76

  irradiated, 301, 307

  knowledge of food sources, 53, 313

  labels, 112, 113, 125–126, 185,
245–246, 248, 311, 343

  lacto-fermented, 76, 81, 318

  processed, 251–252

  protein content of, 345–346

  raw, 77, 81, 312

  as remedy (Hippocrates), 121

  sample menus, 321–325

foreign proteins, 58

Framingham Study, 85, *94*

France, dietary fats and heart
disease, 87

Franken-foods, 34–35

free glutamic acid, *see* MSG
(monosodium glutamate)

free-radicals

  blood glucose and, 138, 166

  trans fats and, 124

  vigorous exercise and, 159

free-range meats, 52

thyroid function (*continued*)
    iodine deficiency and, 268–269
    longevity and, 223
    soy product effects, 64–65
toxicity, heavy metal, 261, 263, 265,
    287
toxins, fat storage and, 84
trace elements
    absorption of, 260
    colloidal mineral avoidance,
        259–260
    digestion and, 70, 73
    health requirements for, 259
    supplemental sources of, 259–260,
        279, 307, 312, 314
    see also individual elements and
        minerals
training of nervous system, 234
trans fats
    adverse effects of, 123–125, 127, 248
    composition and manufacture of,
        123
    dietary avoidance of, 62, 120,
        245–246
    dietary excess of, 84
    disease processes and, 33, 37–38
    fast food and snack food, 55, 125-
        126, *126*
    metabolism and, 111–112
    see also hydrogenated oils
trans-resveratrol supplements,
    176–177, 226–227
transportation advances, health
    improvements and, 39
trypsin inhibitors, 57, 64

U
ulcers, 71, 75, 77
unsaturated fats, 83–84, 93–94
USDA Food Pyramid, 45–47

V
veganism, 235, 318–319
vegetable oils
    cellular membranes and, 117
    dietary availability and
        consumption of, *35, 36*, 120,
        245–246
    dietary avoidance of, 61, 312
    metabolism and, 111–112
vegetables
    dietary fiber and, 192–193
    juicing, 195–196
    protein content of, 346
vegetarianism
    brain and nervous system health
        and, 235, 256, 257
    healthy diet and, 217, 318–319
    information resources, 341
    pre-historic cultures and, 39
    zinc deficiency and, 261
vinpocetine supplements, 258, 273
vitamin A, 77, 97–98
    balance of nutrients and, 100–102,
        105
    deficiencies, 102
    molecular structure, *98*
vitamin B-1, 175
vitamin B6, 250, 271
vitamin B12
    brain health and, 250–251, 256
    deficiencies of, 235
    digestion and health, 70, 73
    soy products and, 64
    supplements, 330
vitamin C, 262, 263, 330
vitamin D
    balance of nutrients and, 100–102,
        105
    benefits of, 99–100, 192
    blood tests and, 103–105, 314

ABOUT THE AUTHOR

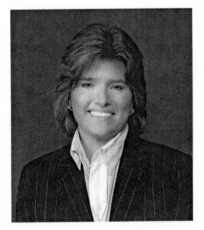

Nora Gedgaudas has a background in diet and nutrition spanning some 25 years and is a widely recognized, respected and sought-after expert in the field.

She is recognized by the Nutritional Therapy Association as a Certified Nutritional Therapist (CNT)/Nutritional Therapy Practitioner (NTP) and is also Board-certified in Holistic Nutrition® through the National Association of Nutritional Professionals (NANP).

Because of her expertise, Nora has appeared as a guest lecturer on radio and television. She is host of her own radio program on Voice America Radio's "Health and Wellness" channel (www.voiceamerica.com) as of May 2009.

Nora served as a trainer for the State of Washington Institute of Mental Health, illuminating nutrition's impact on mental health for State workers at all levels. She maintains a private practice in Portland, Oregon as both a CNT and a Board-Certified clinical Neurofeedback Specialist (CNS).

Breinigsville, PA USA
05 November 2010
248759BV00004B/3/P